BASIC ETHICS

FOR THE

HEALTH CARE PROFESSIONAL

BY

WILLIAM F. MAESTRI
CHARITY HOSPITAL - NEW ORLEANS

with foreword by

Erich K. Lang, M.D.
Director of Radiology, Charity Hospital

Copyright © 1982 by
University Press of America, Inc.℠
P.O. Box 19101, Washington, D.C. 20036

Printed in the United States of America

ISBN: 0-8191-2170-3 (Perfect)
0-8191-2169-X (Case)

Library of Congress Number: 81-40823

This book is dedicated

to all those

at

Charity Hospital

who have made it a

community of

healing and hope.

110973

CONTENTS

FOREWARD

The rapid technoligic development in the health
sciences has lead to the formation of well-defined sub-
specialty areas of learning in the para-medical sciences. The nursing profession carried the responsibility for para-medical and nursing duties almost exclus-
ively through the 1920's and, to some degree, until
World War II. Technological advances in laboratory
medicine and particularly radiology created a need for
dedicated specialists in the early years, the laboratory technologist and the radiologic technologist.
Formal training for these para-medical sub-specialities
was quite brief; the massive impact of expanded technology, however, resulted in an appropriately expanded
training program.

The advent of megavoltage therapy, particle ac-
celerators, ultrasonography, computed axial tomography
and radionuclide imaging have expanded the body of
knowledge to a degree which caused the emergence of
sub-specialty technologists in radiation therapy, ultrasonography, nuclear medicine and, as of late, computed tomography.

Rapid technologic development and expansion in any
field has a profound impact on the prevailing working
conditions and the code of ethics. While the litera-
ture has kept abreast with technologic developments and
has provided the radiologic technologist with a pleth-
ora of scientific and technical informations in all of
the developing sub-specialities of radiologic technology, there has been no concerted effort in the past decade to update basic ethic concepts germaine to this
profession.

Father Maestri's book on basic ethics for the radiologic technologist and other para-medical personnel
offers a superb and timely contribution in this important area. The complexity of interaction of health
care team with the community has caused expansion of
curricula in para-medical fields to include an obliga-
tory course on medical ethics. Father Maestri's book
provides a ready syllabus and reference source for this
type of introductory course.

The discussions on medico-legal responsibility and
confidentiality included in this excellent treatise

as well as the basic presentation of fundamentals and principles of ethics and care offer the student and instructor alike an up-to-date resume of prevailing concepts. The increasing complexity in the relationship of radiologic technologists to physicians, hospital administration and the community demands a keen understanding of the medico-legal basis of medical practice, the rights of the individual patient and the responsibilities of the health care profession toward the community. Father Maestri's book addresses these problems and provides the student with much critical information.

Erich K. Lang, M.D.
Professor and Chairman
Department of Radiology, LSU Medical Center
Professor of Radiology, Tulane School of Medicine
Director, Department of Radiology, Charity Hospital

INTRODUCTION

Technology is one of the most visible aspects of our everyday life. It is hard to imagine one day without the use of technological gadgets. From the alarm clock that wakes us, to the micro-wave oven that heats our frozen food, to the car that carries us to work, to the electric blanket that warms us at night, we are surrounded by a fabricated world. It is equally hard to imagine any of us coming to understand just how these trinkets work. In effect, we are users of technology without possessing the necessary working knowledge of such technologies. This "use only" approach to our fabricated everyday world evokes in us feelings of alienation and powerlessness. When our machines break we must call in the expert. The expert is the new highpriest who possesses the special gnosis (knowledge) that can deliver us from technological frustration. To be without such knowledge is to be vulnerable and open to manipulation. We do not know for sure that the television must be taken to the shop for repair. We remain skeptical, but helpless, when the mechanic informs us that the carburetor needs to be replaced. Such examples of technological frustration and impotence could be multiplied ad infinitum. The main point is this: it is not enough to use technology, one must also come to understand that which one uses. Most especially, one must always question the human ends (values) towards which technology is being applied. Technology cannot be an end in itself, but a means to some human end. The agenda, that is, the ends for which technology is used, is structured by values which determine the who, what, when, and how much of technology. The greatest danger that faces modern humankind in its relationship to technology is an uncritical and taken-for-granted approach. Too often we become aware of technology only when it fails to deliver the goods or services promised. The awesome power of the automobile fails to grasp our attention until it does not start. The same can be said for the light bulb, the air-conditioner, and the countless other machines that structure our everyday life. This taken-for-grantedness is a powerful statement to just how pervasive and ingrained technology has become.

The presence of technology is nowhere more profound and spectacular than in the sphere of modern medical care. Modern medical technology is both a blessing

and a curse. Modern medicine allows us to live longer
with a quality of life that is unsurpassed in the history of humankind. There has been a drastic reduction
in the rate of infant mortality and childhood diseases.
Trauma and sickness that once claimed us and our loved
ones no longer hold sway. Modern medicines, so-called
"wonder drugs", have greatly eliminated or controlled
diseases that once killed large segments of the population. The advent of organ transplants have extended
the lives and restored others to complete wholeness
(eye and kidney, not to mention heart, transplants).
New methods of nutrition and pre- and post- natal care
have done much to insure good health during the forma-
tive years of life. Physicians and various allied
health professionals have done much in the field of
preventive medicine to stop disease before it starts,
or at least, to lessen its effects.

These spectacular successes have a tendency to
blind us to the more troubling aspects of modern medical technology. What now naws at the consciousness and
conscience of the men and women who comprise the "long
white line", and the thoughtful citizenry as well, are
issues of an ethical sort: genetic engineering, abortion, human experimentation and transplant, allocation
of scarce resources and social justice, are but a few.
The specter of Karen Ann Quinlan haunts us all. Death,
once upon a time in those "good ole days", was so easy
to define, or at least declare. One felt a pulse, lis-
tened for a heartbeat, or looked for breath marks on a
mirror. Anyone who happened along knew death when they
saw, heard, or felt it. Even when the physician was
called in to confirm what everyone knew, he performed
pretty much the same tests as the lay person. However,
all that has changed. The waters have become more tur-
bulent and the clear markings are no longer so clear.
Death is not all that easy to define anymore. Death
has been localized in the brain, the heart and bodily
fluids, or some combination thereof (Harvard Medical
School). States have legislated various statutes concerning death. More and more, families, physicians,
and ultimately the courts are being asked to decide
when the "plug can be pulled" and when death can be of-
ficially recognized. Medical technology has exacted a
price on us all.

Technology has drastically restructured our social
and moral world. In many ways our technological know-
how has outdistanced our ethical wisdom. The formation
of an ethic which serves to guide everyday decisions

and help future generations to cope with change usually results from an abundance of time. That is, until fairly recently, there was a sufficient time-lag between significant changes. This time-lag allòws a society to reflect on the enduring problems that must be met and formulate reasonable solutions and mechanisms for coping. Today, however, such a time-lag is missing. The rate of technological change throws us into what Alvin Toffler has termed "Future Shock". There is an absence of sufficient time for a society, or particular group within a society (such as the medical community), to formulate adequate responses and exhibit the necessary adaptive behavior for survival and growth. We are involved in what might be termed a "Technological Catch-22". On the one hand, life is unthinkable without the technological presence we have come to expect as part of our birthright. And yet, much of our technological progress is viewed as a threat to our freedom and dignity.

The presence of technology and machines are the overwhelming visible reality of the radiologic technologist. There is a "clear and present danger" that the human factor will be canceled out or covered over in the demands of the everyday hospital routine. There is always a danger that the patient will cease to be a person and will come to be viewed only as an object of a hospital number and/or a given radiologic routine. When the patient ceases to be encountered as a person and is viewed only as an object the result is dehumanization and brutalization. Not only is the patient robbed of his or her humaness, but the technologist as well ceases to be a human being contributing to the care of the patient. The technologist becomes alienated and is nothing more than an extension of some impersonal, technological process. The technologist is first and foremost a person who happens to be a technologist, not a technologist who happens to be a human being. It is all too easy for the technologist to become subsumed under the imperatives of technological precision at the cost of real human healing or wholeness. What is demanded of the technologist is everyday vigilance concerning the quality of care extended to each patient.

The radiologic technologist is a vital member of the health care community. The technologist is in a position of knowledge and power. This does not, however, guarantee that the technologist will respond with corresponding wisdom or human care. Such knowledge and

power should call forth from the technologist a deep
respect for the patient. With all knowledge comes
power: control of our destiny and that of others.
What is crucial is to develop a virtuous character,
that is, a willingness to do what is in the best interest of the patient. Ours is a society which does not
easily tolerate one who claims to be sick. The claim-
ing of the role and status of "sick person" is often
viewed with suspicion and even hostility. American society is structured around hard work, achievement, and
competition. The one who is sick is excused from pro-
ducing and consuming. The sick person does not contribute, quite the contrary, the sick person is a drain
on our economy. Furthermore, the major thrust of the
advertising establishment is directed to the young and
"beautiful people". A great deal of money is invested
in the "Pepsi Generation" and their consumer taste.
No society so structured can afford to be too tolerant
toward the sick. This is doubly true when the sick are
also poor. These negative feelings must not be denied
or repressed. They should be acknowledged and "educa-
ted" so as to be constructively dealt with. If we ignore or, out of embarassment and guilt, deny them they
will not go away. Such feelings will only be turned
inward and be experienced as depression. It is essential in the growth and motivation of the technologist
to deal with feelings, most especially the negative
ones. The best interest of the patient will be most
effectively served through a complete program of education - the technical as well as our ethical and emotional makeup.

The radiologic technologist as a vital member of
the health care community is concerned primarily with
the care of each patient. The technologist owes his or
her status to the fact that one possesses a special
form of knowledge. With all knowledge comes increased
responsibility. There is an urgent need today to make
technology work for humankind, not for humankind to
work for technology. In recent times, those who are
the guardians of such knowledge and power have been under great pressure to account for their stewardship.
Those in the medical profession have come under increased analysis. In many ways this is a good thing.
However, this is not always easy, especially in an ep-
och in which many of the traditional values and beliefs
of our society have been declared obsolete. Never before has the ethical discourse been needed; yet, never
before has such discourse been so hard to come by. The
foregoing text is an attempt to provide some much

needed reflection on the place and function of ethics in the modern hospital setting.

An introduction should serve as a signal to the reader of the comming attractions as well as the biases and prejudices of the author. First, the subjective signals. I attended and graduated from the School of Radiologic Technology at Charity Hospital in New Orleans (1967-1969). I have turned in my white coat for a black suit and white collar. I am a Catholic priest with the Archdiocese of New Orleans and teach philosophy at the college seminary (St. Joseph Seminary College). For the past three years, I have had the privilege of teaching medical ethics to student technologists at Charity Hospital. This book will no doubt express a given tradition, Catholic Christian, and a given experience, Charity Hospital. However, what follows hopefully meets the needs of all men and women who each day serve the sick as technologists and para-medical professionals. The issues transcend religious traditons and a given hospital setting.

The book will address five (5) major areas of ethical concern: Chapter one will discuss the fundamentals of ethics and offer a brief word about the history and nature of ethical discourse. Chapter two will be devoted to explaining care as the norm which structures the technologist relationship to the patient. Chapter three will offer a brief, but necessary, word about the legal aspects of radiologic technology and the need for confidentiality in the technologist-patient relationship. Chapter four will center on the radiologic technologist and the importance of healthy interpersonal relationships within the hospital community. And finally, chapter five will examine the technologist as moral agent.

A final introductory word seems in order concerning what this book is intended to do, and more importantly, not intended to do. This book is not a blueprint and exact guide for every situation that the technologist will face in the everyday demands of hospital life. No text can make the technologist an ethically sensitive and humanly responsive person. Ethics is not magic and no course can transform one into modern-day Albert Schwietzers. This text does not presume to dictate to each hospital setting what can and should be done. Each school and staff must apply these reflections to their own context. In other words, this book is a first step which invites each hospital community to add "flesh to these bones". Having said what the text is not, we must say what it is: This book in basic ethics is an attempt to enable the radiologic technologist to do some serious thinking about technology and human values. Such an attempt is modest and humble, but these are the paths to truth. This book is directed to the radiologic technologist in particular, however, it can be applied to the wider community of para-professional staff. The text itself is not long and purposefully free of technical terminology . This was done in order to make the text highly adaptive to various hospital and school seetings. Also a large text can give the impression that between the covers of the book are all the answers. However, very often it is the questions that are the most important and exciting. If this text can provide some illumination and evoke some questions it will have fulfilled its function.

This book owes its origin and completion to countless people. My teachers at Charity Hospital gave me an early sensitivity to the human needs present in all medicine. I owe a great debt to the patients with whom I have worked and hopefully helped. Naturally, I am indebted to my students who have patiently struggled with me in coming to think more clearly and deeply about such issues. A special word of gratitude is extended to Anthony Rossi, R.T., Ralph Gutierrez, R.T., Charles Nice, M.D., Charles Hoskins, T.T. and Arthur LaPorte, R.T. Gratitude is expressed to Ana L. Garcia who cheerfully typed this manuscript. Finally, this book is dedicated to all who have devoted their lives to the art of healing.

William F. Maestri
New Orleans, 1980

CHAPTER I

THE FUNDAMENTALS OF ETHICS

Once upon a time ethics as a discipline was held in high esteem. However, like so many of the once valued aspects of life, ethics has fallen into ill repute. Today ethics is viewed as mere opinion, personal taste, etiquette, social convention, or a relative expression of cultural values that differ from culture to culture. In other words, there are no lasting, objective values by which we can determine right and wrong behavior. In addition, ethics has come to be viewed as a limitation on one's freedom and an ideology used by the powerful to control the powerless. Also, ethics demands that we believe, trust, and hope in that which is beyond us. Viet Nam, Watergate, and various political scandals have increased our skepticism and elevated cynicism and suspicion to predominant attitudes. In other words, it is harder to believe today. All of these factors make the talk about ethics seem harder to believe today. All of these factors make the talk about ethics seem like a "noisy gong and clanging cymbal". Yet, it is just because such a climate of ethical negation is so pervasive that the need for doing ethics is so important. The absence of ethics and moral values as a guide for individual and social behavior does not increase our freedom; quite the contrary, without ethics and moral values life becomes "short, brutish, and hard". Man is the values animal. Our everyday vocabulary is loaded with moral and values terminology: right-wrong; good-bad; virtue-vice; like-dislike; praise-blameworthy. To deny or attempt to eliminate ethics is to cover over an essential element of our humanity. To be human is to be involved in the morals game. The issue is not whether we <u>want</u> to play, but rather <u>how</u> shall we play. We need to ask: Just what is ethics?

Ethics is the art and science which seeks to determine the rightness and wrongness of human behavior according to some norm or standard. Before developing this definition further it is of the utmost importance to keep in mind that ethics is both and art and a science. In many ways the art-science nature of ethics parallels the art-science nature of medicine and radiologic technology. The parallel bewteen ethics and medicine is as old as Aristotle (384 BC-322 BC) and just as valid today as when he first suggested it. In

Aristotle's monumental ethical work, <u>Nicomachean Ethics</u>, he draws the following similarities between doing ethics and medicine: (1) ethics and medicine are both practical activities. The goal of each is the proper action by an individual directed to the attainment of some end. For ethics one seeks to achieve the good or praiseworthy. For medicine one seeks to heal the sick. (2) Ethics and medicine are both concerned with individual cases and the circumstances which contribute to the uniqueness of each situation. One needs to know both the general principles and how to apply those principles to each individual case. General principles of ethics and medicine take on meaning when they are applied to the concrete situations that confront us. (3) Ethics and medicine are both concerned with the well-being of the whole person: mind, body, and spirit or soul. Ethics seeks to describe and prescribe human behavior in view of the person as a whole or unified entity. Ethics pays careful attention to what the sciences and arts have to say about the human person and his or her possibilities. There has been in recent times a revival in medicine which seeks to heal the patient, not merely on a physical level, but seeks healing in a holistic way. Healing involves the physical and spiritual dimensions of the person. (4) Ethics and medicine do not yield precise, absolute, and unchanging knowledge. Ethics and medicine are organismic disciplines, that is, they are always growing and changing in light of new insights and techniques. This can be very frustrating for those who seek certainty and security. Such is not to be had with ethics and medicine. Yet, this is the real excitement and adventure of these disciplines. Ethics and medicine are disciplines of high adventure which demand we learn to live securely with our insecurities. Ethics and medicine offer to those who accept their invitation a life of zest that comes from all true learning and growth.

There are three important elements in our definition of ethics that deserve further explanation: ethics as art, as science, and ethics as related to some norm or standard of behavior. Ethics is an art in that ethics requires more than the use of our intellect. Ethics requires that we use all of our faculties in determining what ought to be done in a given situation. Ethics involves most especially the use of the creative imagination in selecting a proper course of action. Our intellect, memory, and imagination are required for the development of truly human moral values. Ethics is art in that we must be sensitive to our feelings, every day experiences, intuitions, and respect the traditions of the various groups to which we belong. In this way, ethics as an art touches us at the depth of our being. Ethics is more than a clear and neat formula which yields a detailed course of action. As an art, ethics demands that we develop a "feel" or sensitivity for human acts and values that help promote a more humane environment. Ethics like art is not totally explainable. There is always more to ethical analysis than we are able to articulate. Finally, this aspect of "necessary incompleteness" in all our ethical analysis should evoke in us a sense of humility. That is, our ethical judgments should not become ethically judgmental. The realization that our values and courses of action are always tentative should evoke in us a tolerance for others and a willingness to learn from the experience and insights of others.

Not only is ethics an art it is also a science. Ethics is not just a matter of taste, good feeling, or doing one's own thing. Ethics is like science in that ethics sights the facts, assesses the circumstances, and studies the empirical data relevant to a given situation. Ethics is not done in a vacuum, but is most sensitive to the need for gathering information. If one ignores the necessity for empirical fact gathering, then ethical judgments will be mere sentiment. The goal of ethics as a science is to render objective judgments. This goal is an ideal which is never completely reached. However, it must always remain the operative ideal in our judgments and actions. In saying that ethics as a science seeks impartial, objective judgments, we are not saying that one seeks passionless truth. Ethics is an activity which involves us as human beings in our completeness, that is, mind and feelings, intellect and will. Ethics demands that we become involved and be concerned. The greatest danger to the doing of ethics is apathy or a lack of feeling or passion for that which we seek to preserve or change. Apathy in ethical analysis is often hidden under the mask of an "ideal, impartial spectator" who wants to be "above it all". Ethics demands however, that we gather the evidence, as in any science, and the evidence is gathered in the real, everyday world where we live, move, and have our being. In effect, to do ethics is to do the work of the scientist, the artist, and the serious professional.

All ethical systems are grounded in a norm or standard which serves to guide the person in determining

the goodness and badness of an act. In general, a norm
is a rule, or standard, or value by which we measure,
rate, or judge an act or achievement. Norms are not
confined to the area of morality. For example, in
baseball the player who bats .300 or the pitcher who
wins twenty games has a very good year. The student
who earns a C is considered average. In the area of
ethical analysis a norm functions in much the same way.
A moral norm is a standard, rate, or primary value
which indicates what behavior is worthy of praise (virtue) and which acts are to be avoided (vice). Most
ethical systems agree on what is acceptable behavior
and what acts should be avoided. The real difference
between ethical systems arise when one discusses the
norms or standards by which one judges behavior. In
other words, the difference that separate various systems of ethics centers around the reasons for the ap-
proval and disapproval of various acts. Throughout the
history of Western moral philosophy three systems have
predominated: Utilitarianism, ethical formalism, and
natural law ethics. A brief word about each of these
systems will be helpful in introducing the student to
the Western ethical heritage. Also, the student will
be introduced to the norms or primary values that have
concerned moral theorists.

UTILITARIANISM. This moral philosophy was formulated by two eighteenth and nineteenth century British
moral philosophers: Jeremy Bentham (1748-1832) and
John Stuart Mill (1806-1873). British utilitarianism
is the most influential school of ethics in the history
of British philosophy and has had great influence in A-
merica. Utilitarianism is the philosophical approach
to moral behavior which holds that the ultimate goodness and badness of an act depends on the consequences
produced. The more pleasurable the consequences the
greater the happiness, and therefore, the more virtuous
the act. By contrast, one should seek to avoid pain
and subsequent unhappiness. The utilitarian ethics is
centered around the belief that happiness, pleasure,
and virtue are interrelated. All actions which produce happiness are pleasurable and praiseworthy.

We can summarize the essential elements of utilitarianism in the following way:

1. Pain and pleasure are the two sovereign mas-
ters which govern the behavior of humankind. The motivation for the doing of certain actions and the re-
fraining from doing others is our desire to attain

4

pleasure and avoid pain.

2. The utilitarian view of human nature is less than optimistic. Man seeks his own pleasure first and foremost and wants to avoid pain at all cost. There is no real altruism or selfless doing good for others. Even our charity is egotistical and self-serving. We do good works in order to feel superior, satisfied, or powerful. This does not mean that we never help others. We must and we do help others, however, this is done in order to insure our own happiness.

3. All moral acts are judged in terms of consequences, that is, the amount of happiness produced. There are no intrinsically right or wrong acts. Acts become right or wrong in view of the consequences produced. An act which produces happiness is good; one which produces pain is bad. For example, the eating of a well prepared meal is very pleasurable and therefore good. However, the eating of the same meal becomes bad if done by one who must adhere to a strict diet. The eating of a high sugar meal may cause one great pain and therefore be bad.

4. Utilitarianism ultimately rests on a calculus, that is the ability to measure the amount of happiness produced by a given course of action or competing courses of action. The Utilitarian is concerned with determining the amount or quantity of pleasure produced. In this way the utilitarian hopes to make ethics an exact science. Bentham indicates in his work, Introduction to the Principles of Morals and Legislation, the following go into measuring the amount of happiness (pleasure produced): intensity, duration, certainty, purity, the extent to which others share my pleasure, and the reasonable expectation for other pleasures to follow from my course of action.

5. John Stuart Mill in his great work, Utilitarianism, amends the initial utilitarian principle of the greatest happiness to be more social in nature. That is, Mill amends the principle to read: "the greatest happiness for the greatest number". Happiness is the ultimate norm of utilitarian morality, but it is not the happiness of the individual agent alone. The greatest happiness must contribute to the greatest number and this is achieved through the use of reason. In addition to this social amendment, Mill also argued for a more qualitative understanding of pleasure. For the most part we live by ordinary, everyday pleasure. Once

in a while we experience moments of rapture and intense pleasure. Human beings, furthermore, seek not only sensual or physical pleasure, but we seek pleasures of the mind and the fulfillment of our creative, artistic needs. Both the physical and intellectual (spiritual) must be satisfied.

CRITIQUE OF UTILITARIANISM

Utilitarianism is a moral philosophy which can be criticized on a number of grounds. Among the more salient criticisms advanced are the following:

1. On a methodological basis it is difficult, if not impossible, to measure with a reasonable degree of accuracy the amount of pleasure yielded by a given act.

2. It is not always possible to predict the consequences of a given act. Many of our actions have what is termed unforeseeable consequences. Our best plans and most careful calculations at times simply do not work out. What we think may produce the most pleasure may in fact turn out to be anything but pleasurable. Should we be declared immoral in spite of our best intentions and most careful preparations? One would think not.

3. Utilitarianism is not the first philosophical system to propose happiness as the end goal which we seek. Aristotle and St. Thomas Aquinas also believed that all behavior was directed toward the attainment of happiness. However, what is particular to the utilitarians is the equating happiness with pleasure. Aristotle believed that happiness was achieved through the proper development of one's rational nature. St. Thomas believed man could only be truly happy through a participation in the mind of God (Beatific or Blessed Vision). Can happiness really be equated with pleasure? Are not there cases in which we must suffer for a greater good? For example, an operation involves some pain and suffering, yet it is quite necessary in order to live. One may have to suffer much for a friend or loved one, yet one does so willingly in the name of love.

4. Related to the difficulty of equating happiness with pleasure is the failure to define pleasure in a general or universal way. In other words, pleasure becomes a subjective expression of one's own taste.

6

What makes me happy may not make you happy and vice
versa. Happiness becomes in the final analysis an em
ty term.

5. The utilitarian principle of the "greatest
happiness for the greatest number" can be used to jus
tify the sacrificing of the individual to achieve
group interest. For example, such a principle could
used to sanction medical experimentation on a patient
with or without the person's consent. In the name of
the public good or for the benefit of future generations the rights of the individual could be taken awa
Such a principle could be very dangerous if applied
literally to control populations in prisons and menta
hospitals. Their populations could be used simply as
means to achieve a social goal; in this, a serum is e
fective. The goal or end is noble; however, the mear
are questionable to say the least. In effect, the er
does not justify any means.

The above critique is not said so as to leave th
impression that utilitarianism is totally without val
dity. The enduring contribution of the utilitarian
perspective is its demand that we take human experier
seriously. The utilitarian view calls us to pay atte
tion to what we do and exercise responsibility in the
acts we perform. The utilitarians are reminding us
that our actions have real consequences for ourselves
and others. We cannot act with insensitivity or disr
gard for others. Simply put, for every action there
a reaction, and the reactions or consequences we produce indicate the kind of human being we are becoming

ETHICAL FORMALISM. The philosopher we most
closely associate with this moral perspective is the
German thinker Immanuel Kant (1724-1804). Kant was
disturbed by the attacks on science delivered by British philosopher David Hume (1711-1776). Hume denied
the principle of causality and claimed that cause and
effect was nothing more than a psychological habit of
the mind. There is no necessary relationship of caus
ality in the world. There is no intrinsic causal relationship between event (a) and (b). The fact that
(b) follows (a) is mere habit and may not occur in th
future. In addition, Kant was disturbed that religio
was being attacked by philosophers of a rationalistic
bent and also by scientists who considered religion t
be nothing more than superstition. Also Kant rejecte

7

the Utilitarian emphasis on consequences and sought to
ground morality in the norm of duty to the law. For
Kant, morality is a deontalogical discipline, that is,
moral behavior is judged according to some principle or
value by which one ought to act or avoid from acting.
The Utilitarian view is what we term teleological, that
is, the rightness and wrongness of an act is determined
by the consequences and not by a given set of principles. Kant's moral philosophy is contained chiefly in
two works: <u>Critique of Practical Reason</u> and <u>Fundamen-
tal Principles of the Metaphysic of Morals</u>. Let us
now examine Kant's view of the moral life.

Kant believes that each act is moral if and only
if that act results from a good will. By a good will
Kant means one that acts, not from selfish interest or
egoism, but from duty. Not only must one act according
to duty as prescribed by the law, but one must intend
to do the act because it is commanded by the law. A
good will involves both the act and the intention. An
act is good not because of its consequences, but because of respect for the law. For Kant a good will
which obeys the moral law out of a sense of duty alone
endures and has moral value. As Kant says, "a good
will would shine like a jewel for its own sake as
something which has its full value in itself".

The question naturally arises: what is the law
for which we must show respect and will to do? It is
not any particular set of laws as such, but rather, it
is the idea or concept of law itself. This respect for
law as a pure concept is what Kant calls the "Categorical imperative". By this Kant means, "I ought never to
act except in such a way that I can also will that my
maxim should become a universal law". In other words,
any course of action that I freely choose must be ap-
plicable to everyone else regardless of circumstances
and without exception. What I do must be an example
and not an exception. Kant believed that he had set
morality on an objective plane. The categorical imperative is formal, that is, it lacks specific content or
a given set of actions. As a responsible moral agent
I must fill in the given course of action to be done
for evaluation. The categorical imperative is universal; every act must be purposed for everyone else to do
without exception. In effect, the categorical imperative proclaims the moralequality of persons. What is
good for the proverbial goose is good for the gander"

Kant understands the uniqueness and greatness of

the human being to be found in one's rationality. The nobility of reason demands that I be moral and responsible for what I do. In addition to requiring that any individual acts become universal laws, Kant adds a second, and crucial element, to the moral life: "One ought never treat the self or another as a means only to some end. Each person and the self must be treated as an end in themselves." The self and other human beings are not things or objects to be manipulated by our calculations and desires. Each person possesses dignity and worth beyond their utility or market value. The nobility of the person is grounded in one's nature as a free and rational being who is called to the moral life. To treat myself or another as a pure means to achieve some end, however good, is not morally permissable. Therefore, the two basic principles in Kant's formalism are: the willing of one's actions to be morally binding on everyone. And secondly, the respect for persons which demands we never use others or oneself as a means only.

Is the moral law, which binds all of us, imposed by the church, state, or family? No. The moral law is never imposed from outside, but is something which I impose on myself. The freedom of the will demands that I accept the moral law as my own. Such an exercise of our free will further highlights our dignity as rational beings. The existence of the moral law, says Kant, is evidenced by our free will, immortality of the soul, and the existence of God. If we are not free then morality makes no sense whatsoever. Each of us is limited and can only approximate the moral law in its perfection. However, this does not call us to passive acceptance of our imperfection. We must continually strive to reach perfection. Kant believed that such perfection is only attained in some after life existence (heaven if you will). And finally since we have some basic notion of the good and the moral, however imperfect, there must be a perfection of the good and the moral. Kant believes that it is God alone who is the ultimate fulfillment of both.

CRITIQUE OF KANTIAN FORMALISM

There is much to commend Kant's moral philosophy. However, before we highlight its contributions, three limitations need to be mentioned.

1. The motivation for all moral behavior is duty,

and only duty. This absolutizing of duty denies the presence of other motivational factors. For example, is the relationship between teacher and student, parent and child, doctor and patient, only structured by a sense of duty? How many times does one go beyond duty and make tremendous sacrifices, not out of a sense of duty, but from a deep feeling of love and genuine concern? Acts in which one sacrifices oneself for the good of others cannot be commanded by duty or ordered by the law. Acts of human nobility do not come from the letter of the law or duty, but from the spirit which reaches beyond the law. The law cannot command one to offer a relative or stranger a kidney. Such sacrifice comes from that which is beyond duty. However, to do such a thing as donate one's kidney is a-moral, that is, an act which cannot claim to be moral. Such a conclusion seems rather inhuman.

2. Kant sought to escape what he believes is the relativism of the utilitarian position, that is, the rightness or wrongness of an act depends on the consequences. However, Kant falls into subjectivism by making the motive of the moral agent determinitive of the moral quality of any act. In effect, whether any act is right or wrong depends on the motive of the person performing the act. Just like the utilitarian position, no act is right or wrong in itself (intrinsic), but each act becomes moral in light of the motive of the agent.

3. Kant correctly emphasizes the need for a free will if one is to speak about morality. It will be remembered that Kant answered the question as to who imposed the moral law by saying that one imposes it on oneself. No law is binding which I have not chosen for myself. In other words, there can be no genuine freedom as long as one is placed under a law imposed by others. But why is this so? There is no necessary contradiction between a free will and a law that is commanded by another. Kant leaves us with a will that is answerable only to itself. There is no real duty or obligation in such a system. For I am duty-bound to accept only that which I freely choose. But I am totally free to accept any which as long as I postulate it for everyone (categorical imperative). In effect, all authentic obligation seems to be swept aside.

As in the case with utilitarianism there is great value in Kant's moral philosophy. Of special :

10

signifcance are the following two aspects:

1. Kant forcefully reminds us of the importance of doing one's duty and the need for law if social life is not to degenerate into a state of "all against all". This is of great importance in an age such as ours in which the ethical imperative is often "doing one's own thing", "life is to be enjoyed", and "do it if it feels good". Kant reminds us that there are great and small aspects of our life that demand we do things for no other reason than it is our duty. Kant calls us to transcend our feelings and do what is required. If we take Kant's categorical imperative seriously, act so as your behavior can be a universal law, one can only shudder to think what would happen if we followed our feelings alone, or merely did something because it felt good.

2. Of special importance to those in the medical profession is Kant's injunction that one must never treat the self or others as a means only, but always as an end. The rise of new technologies and new experiments must never be allowed to turn the patient into an object or means in order to achieve some medical end. The need for free and informed consent must always be carried out in an effort to protect the dignity of the individual. No end or goal, however good or noble or beneficial, can ever transcend the worth of the individual person. In a century which has witnessed so much brutalization and violation of human rights, the need to value each person can never be over-emphasized.

NATURAL LAW ETHICS. The Father of the Western philosophical tradition, Socrates (470-399B.C.), used to ask his students, "Are things good because we desire them, or should we desire them because they are good?" A great many today would select the first part of Socrates' question. Since the time of Rene Descartes (1596-1650), the so-called founder of modern philosophy, we usually answer questions and select values on a subjective basis. Therefore, the goodness of something is derived from the fact that I desire it, and not because it is good in itself (objectively good). However, the answer suggested by Socrates and the vast majority of traditional philosophers is in the opposite direction. Goodness is an objective quality that does not depend on human willing or desire. Socrates believed (along with Plato and Aristotle as well) that we desire a thing because it is good in itself. The good, from the perspective of Socrates and those who follow in his footsteps, is something objective and cannot be reduced to consequences or the autonomous will. The natural law theory of ethics would certainly agree with Plato that goodness, truth, and beauty are objective realities and not human desire.

The natural law theory of ethics is most closely associated with Aristotle (384-322 B.C.) and St. Thomas Aquinas (1225-1274 A.D.). The Catholic moral tradition has been the leading proponent and exponent of natural law ethics as formulated by St. Thomas Aquinas. Although the association of natural law with religion is quite strong, it should be kept in mind that the origin of natural law is with a group of early pagan Greek philosophers called Stoics. The Stoics beleived that there was no distinction between physical law and moral laws. The proper use of reason enables one to know about the world and what one ought to do in the moral realm of everyday life. The natural law is part of the very nature of all reality, including a law written into the heart of each person. This law informs the person what must be done if one is to become what one already is - a human being. The right use of reason was needed if one was to know the natural law. Even though the law was written into one's nature, the human being is free to turn from the dictates of reason and nature, and follow one's passions or desires.

Natural law ethics had a great appeal for Christian philosophers and teachers since it offered an objective basis for morality - the nature of man which is universal, uniform, and a-historical. That is, the nature of man is a constant throughout history and remains the same from culture to culture. To be human is to have certain fundamental needs (spiritual/intellectual, social, biological) and a unique faculty which enables man to be superior to the rest of nature - the rational soul or intellect. Man is the thinking animal and in the proper use of reason man becomes what he is meant to be - a rational animal. From such a perspective, the moral life is not the product of subjective willing, cultural values, or consequences, but is part of the very nature and structure of reality. The moral life is the same for all human beings. The Christian tradition could not accept the Stoic understanding of natural law in toto. The Christian tradition responded to the question - Who gives this law? - by introducing God as Creator and law-giver. The Christian tradition blends the Bible with Greek philosophy. God creates (Genesis) and, in creating, God has determined by laws

12

the end or goal to which all creation is drawn. The
most comprehensive formulation of natural law ethics
was done by St. Thomas Aquinas in his monumental work
Summa Theologica (to be specific, Summa Theologica, I-
II pp. 90-108 "The Treatise on Law"). According to St.
Thomas the natural law is part of a fourfold system of
laws. St. Thomas called these laws eternal, divine,
natural, and positive. The eternal law is the law that
is present in the mind of God and therefore unknowable
to the finite mind of man. This eternal law is God's
pure will or desire. How is man to know what God wants?
The divine law is the will of God as revealed in the
Scriptures and the life of Jesus. Through revelation
man can know what God wants (Ten Commandments). But
suppose one never heard of Jesus or the Christian God?
Suppose one was born before Jesus came or in a part of
the world that remains untouched by missionary efforts?
Each human being can still know what God desires through
the natural law. The natural law is the minimum requirements placed on all human beings by the very fact
they are human. So the Hindu in India and the native
in the deepest recesses of the jungle can still serve
God by following the inborn inclination of one's nature.
Through the proper use of reason anyone can come to
know what is required in order to be a moral human being. This knowledge of the natural law is not an all
or nothing affair. While we all have, by nature, some
inborn understanding of what is required of a human being, our knowledge of the natural law needs to be deep-
ened through constant study and discipline. Finally,
man is by nature a social animal and requires the com-
pany of his fellows. No man is to live without others;
in other words in society, there must be a system of
man-made laws which promote peace, harmony, and justice. The positive laws are those laws that are man-
made and result from the needs of the community. The
stopping at a red light is an example of the positive
law. St. Thomas says that a society cannot formulate
any sort of law and make it morally binding. Positive
laws are moral and binding when they conform to reason
and are in agreement with the divine law. The laws of
slavery are immoral and unnatural since they treat the
human being as if he were a piece of property or thing.
Slavery denies the very essence of man by treating him
only as a means to some economic or social end.

CRITIQUE OF NATURAL LAW ETHICS

        As in the case of utilitarianism and ethical for-
malism, natural law ethics has much to commend it as

well as some serious drawbacks. First the limitations of which three seem significant.

1. The key terms of natural law ethics, person, nature, and essence, are holdovers from a Greek culture and historical period that no longer speaks to our contemporary experience and understanding. These terms were understood in a fixed and unchanging way. The nature of man hss not changed since he first appeared on earth. However, such a view contradicts the evidence of science and evolution. Today we are much more aware of changes and flux. Of special importance is modern man's sensitivity to various historical periods and their influence on what was held to be true and good. This historical consciousness reminds us of the temporality and limitations of our beliefs and values. Today reality is a process and to be alive is to know change and experience flux.

2. Even if one accepts there is a natural law this does not really solve the problem of means in order to achieve the goal of our nature. To say that one must follow correct reason remains insensitive to the differences that exist between people who in good faith disagree about just what is reasonable and what is proper. Also, people have differences concerning just which acts are in accordance with one's nature or the natural law. If natural law is objective and universal, one would expect there to be agreement between those acts which are in conformity with one's nature and the means used to reach the natural ends.

3. Many critics believe that natural law is insensitive to circumstances of the individual person. In other words, natural law become natural legalism. By this critics mean that the human component in ethics becomes ignored and only the law is of value. However, many would say that the law is meant to serve man and not man the law. The law must not become an end in itself, but always a mean to some human end. The law should serve man and aid in the enrichment of life and the growth of the person and society.

Natural law ethics has a long and well-respected history, and not without good reason. Three of the more important contributions of the natural perspective are the following:

1. While it is true that we cannot speak about human nature as if it were an absolutely fixed entity,

modern social and biological sciences do allow us to
speak about basic or fundamental human needs and abilities common to man as a species. Psychiatrist Abraham
Maslow (1954) has done much work in studying human
needs that we all have, and these needs exist in a hi-
erarchy: physiological needs, safety, belongingness
and love, esteem, and finally, self-actualization. The
degree to which these needs must be met vary; however,
the basic needs remain constant for all human beings.
In other words, if human nature can be understood in a
more flexible way, then natural law has much to contribute to our understanding of what it means to be moral.

2.   As mentioned previously, critics often accuse
natural law ethics of legalism. However, this ought
not to negate the value and necessity of law. The mere
fact that law can be abused is not a sufficient and
necessary argument for the abolishment of law. No one
would seriously advocate the elimination of medicine
because of the immoral, selfish behavior of some medical personnel. Natural law ethics is an attempt to
place ethics and the moral life on a more objective basis. In an attempt to remove ethics from total subjectivism or cultural relativity, the natural law perspective seeks to ground the moral life in the very nature of man, a nature we all share. In our own age of
moral confusion it is hard not to appreciate such an
attempt.

3.   The natural law perspective reminds us that
the laws of society are not ends in themselves, but are
always subject to review by a higher law - the divine
and eternal law. Such a view can keep a society from
expressing the arrogance and intolerance for others
that we so often have witnessed in this century. Human
laws are limited and imperfect. The State and the
leaders of government are answerable not only to the
people they serve, but from the natural law perspective,
all experience of political power comes under the judgment of God. The belief that we are a nation under God
is very important as an aspect of the American religious and political experience.

SUMMARY

This chapter is the most theoretical in the book.
In it we have attempted to present the most basic concepts of moral philosophy. Furthermore, we have attempted to show how the major Western philosophical
systems have addressed the moral life. The three most

influential moral systems are utilitarianism, Kantian formalism, and natural law ethics. Each system has presented what it believes to be the norm or standard for guiding and judging human conduct. Utilitarianism looks to the consequences. Kantian formalism advocates duty to the moral law and a good will. Finally, the natural law perspective views the moral life as one in which the person follows the dictates of reason. Also, in our discussion we attempted to highlight both the advantages and disadvantages of each system.

This chapter may at first seem to be irrelevant to the concerns of the para-medical professional. However, it is of crucial importance for the medical professional and the well-informed citizen to be aware of our ethical traditions. Such an awareness is crucial in the formulation of our personal and professional codes of conduct. We are not the first generation to struggle with moral issues. Hopefully, we will not be the last. The medical professional must not only be technically proficient, but also morally sensitive.

Having laid the foundation for our ethical discussion, it is now time for us to turn specifically to the medical professional's norm of morality. Chapter two will discuss care as the norm and standard for guiding our everyday behavior in the hospital setting. Care is the value and attitude which is the essential for those who undertake the responsibility of helping the sick and vulnerable members of our society and the human family.

CHAPTER II

THE PRINCIPLE OF CARE

In the not too long ago, ethics was a very minor aspect of the physician's training. In many instances such ethical training had as its goal the development of a good "bedside manner". In other words, ethics was equated with etiquette. The ethical doctor was the polite doctor. However, with the increased presence of technology in medicine, an increased sensitivity of the patient to his or her rights, and the desire on the part of the physicians themselves to receive ethical training in a more comprehensive way, there has been a tremendous explosion of courses and seminars dealing with ethics and medical practice. The emergence of courses in professional and medical ethics has expanded beyond the confines of the hospital and have found their way into graduate and undergraduate colleges and seminaries. No doubt one can call this meteoric rise "just another fad". This is always a danger. Many are attracted to the issues that concern the medical ethicist just because they are new and exciting. If medical ethics as a discipline is not only to survive but grow and make a significant contribution to human knowledge and human care for the patient, it will have to prove its worth like any new kid on the block. Medical ethics will do this to the extent that it demands quality above quantity and does not seek to grow through selling its soul to the spectacular. Medical ethics demands the best of physician, patient, and concerned citizen.

In addition to the concern of the physician and patient for ethical training, society at large is experiencing a deep questioning about values, what constitutes the good life, and moral rules. These questions have become more urgent in recent times with the increased presence of technology in the areas of medicine and biology. Also the dilemmas in medicine and biology that result from this technological presence are no longer merely for an elite few. The television and newspaper have made bio-medical dilemmas part of everyone's cognitive world, for example, the trial of Dr. Kenneth Edelin convicted of manslaughter following the death of a fetus supposedly born alive. The case of Karen Ann Quinlain continues to haunt us. The research done by Boston scientists which suggests a connection between criminality and the discovery of the

17

XYY syndrome. Recent court decisions centering on a-
bortion and the right of individuals and companies to
pattern new forms of life made in the laboratory are a
source of heated debate. The ability to produce life
in a test-tube (in vitro) as with little Louise Brown
in England has caused many to think in terms of a 'new
genesis'. These examples and countless others have
sent shock waves throughout society. The old structures and answers are crumbling under the pressure.
Society is questioning and demanding better answers and
training for those entrusted with such power. Society
is demanding all its professionals in the fields of medicine and biology address these moral issues.

If the physician received little or no formal ethical training beyond the development of medical bedside
etiquette, the para-medical professional received even
less. There are many reasons for this increase in ethical training received by the para-medical professional. Technologists, nurses, and aides are more in contact with the patient on a day to day basis. Secondly,
the educational and professional training of para-medical personnel has greatly increased in all aspects.
Thirdly, the various licensing organizations have done
much to emphasize the need for ethical training as part
of the licensing and certification process (for example, the Association of Registered Radiologic Technologists requires a formal course in ethical principles).
Fourthly, the para-medical fields are now recognized as
professions. With this recognition comes the need for
greater accountability to society and the individual patient each professional serves. Finally, the desire
for ethical training has come from the various professions themselves. Many of the medical professionals
feel a need not only for technical expertise, but also
for formal ethical training. The rise of this desire
for a more comprehensive and formal ethical training
program is a sign of real hope. It is a signal that
medicine as a whole is sensitive to the dilemmas of
new technologies and the new situation in which medicine is being done. The physician and the para-medical
professional are saying that they and the patient requires more than technical and scientific training.
Those dedicated to the healing profession are saying
that in order to be effective in their art more is required than technical competence. There is a need for
both technical and ethical training.

The mere desire for courses in ethics and the fact
that such courses are available does not guarantee that

18

ethical sensitivity will result. The climate of ethical discourse today is not all that clear and, in fact, is quite muddled and confused. The traditional landmarks that once clearly indicated right and wrong no longer hold sway. In many ways we face a more challenging and difficult task than past generations who struggled with moral issues: we are trying to formulate a moral concensus without an agreed upon ethical and civil tradition. The fact that the traditional landmarks of right and wrong have lost their power makes it essential for the communities of the physician and the para-medical to structure a humane ethical theory and practice. The medical community as a whole is presented with a tremendous opportunity to serve and be a pioneer for other professional communities struggling with similar tasks. The medical community is struggling to formulate a set of ethical guidelines which will serve the best interest and healing of the patient and the standards of proper professional training. The alternative to ethical and professional standards established by the medical community is often unpleasant. That is, guidelines and standards will be imposed by the courts or by state and federal legislatures. However, such ethical formulations ought not to come from outside the medical community, but should be developed from within by the entire medical community in dialogue with society at large.

Medicine enjoys a high degree of status in our society. With this status comes the admiration, respect, and monetary rewards of a grateful citizenry. This social reverence and gratitude was not easily won. It was not until the middle of the 19th century that medicine gained a respected place in the social order as a profession. This reverence, not easily won, possesses no written guarantee that it will continue. (In fact, there are signs that the white coat is turning a bit yellow. Voices in our society are becoming vocally desparate in their discontent with the quality and cost of medical care. The recent rise of medically related law suits only adds to an already tense situation. For example, a sign in a California doctor's office read as follows: "Need a physician? Call a lawyer." Such signs of discontent by society are not directed only at the medical establishment. One of the results of the sixties was a general discontent with institutions and authority in general. There is no doubt that medicine is a big institution and weilds considerable power in our everyday lives.) The proliferation of technology in modern medicine has spawned a whole cluster of

related para-medical and professional positions. These
technical professions will be held in high esteem and
regarded accordingly if, and only if, the conduct of
each profession and its individual members merits such
respect. The need to formulate a professional code of
ethics and a set of standards for technical competence
is crucial. The need for an ethical code and standards
for technical competence extends beyond the pragmatic,
utilitarian need of social rewards. Such codes and
standards touch on the crucial question of the kind of
human being that is allowed to participate in the art
of healing. The need for ethical reflections springs
from a desire to live an "examined life" and take responsibility for our actions. Ethical reflection helps
to deepen our sensitivity to the fact that we live in a
world with others and the medical vocation is a call to
live for others as well. In the final analysis the value of ethical reflections was best expressed by Plato:
"For no light matter is at stake (ethics); the question
concerns the very manner in which human life is to be
lived." (The Republic).

In chapter one we spoke about norm and how it
functions in various ethical systems. We said an ethical norm is a standard or rule which guides or morally
informs our actions and values. Not only do various
systems of philosophical ethics have norms, but so do
various groups and organizations. The need to formulate a standard of conduct is crucial for any professional group. The lawyer is bound by the canons of
professional conduct and ethics by the American Bar Association and various local certification authorities.
The physician takes the Hippocratic Oath and is judged
professionally and ethically by local medical boards of
review. The radiologic technologist and other para-
medical professionals need to develop and take seriously a code of ethics and professional conduct. The need
to formulate a norm of conduct and a systematic code of
ethics and standards of professional behavior is crucial. The para-medical professional encounters the patient when the person is most vulnerable, helpless, and
open to manipulation. The greatest sensitivity must be
excercised in relating to the patient in a respectful
manner. Therefore, the norm or standard of ethics
which will serve to guide the para-medical professional's everyday conduct is that of CARE.

What is the principle or norm of care as it relates to the radiologic technologist and the para-professional in general? The principle of care calls for

the utmost respect for the sacredness and dignity of
human life in all its forms and conditions. Most especially, care requires the honoring and valuing of
life when it is in need due to illness or trauma. Care
is the fundamental ethical expression and the court of
final appeal in deciding what actions should and should
not be taken. The principle of care is the essential
motive at work in all of our encounters with the patient. Care demands that we always and in every way do
what is in the best interest of the patient according
to the following criteria: the application of care as
the primary consideration in the particular situation,
adherence to accepted rules and medical practice as
they pertain to our given area of competence and training, and finally, to do everything in our power to protect and promote the bond of loyalty between the patient and the entire hospital community. Furthermore,
care demands that we foster a genuine spirit or attitude of compassion towards the patient and his or her
genuine needs. It must be kept in mind that care is a
general principle which takes on full meaning when it
is applied to the given, real life situation. The
principle of care serves to guide and inform daily conduct. However, no principle or norm can indicate what
the para-medical professional is to do specifically in
each case. No principle can insure automatic, infalli-
ble answers. No norm can excuse the para-medical professional from the responsibility to use his or her
creative intellect and imagination in deciding how best
to practice genuine human care for this patient, in
this situation, and under these circumstances. Care
requires that the medical professional develop the
skills and values of prudence, moral sensitivity, and
be open to learning from one's individual and group
experience.

In proposing the principle of care as the norm for
para-medical professional ethics we are seeking to
place daily medical practice within the Judeo-Christian
tradition. In effect, the professional and ethical behavior of medical personnel are rooted in the living,
on-going experience of our moral heritage. This allows
us to draw on the insights of the past and articulate
standards for more humane conduct in the future. The
principle of care bestows upon the medical community a
history, a memory if you will, that grounds present experience in an on-going story. To be specific, the
principle of care is related to the Jewish experience
of hesed and the Christian experience of agape. Hesed
is a Jewish word derived from the Biblical experience

21

of God's (Yahweh) steadfast fidelity and love for His
people Israel. The hesed of God is a love which is
tender and yet demanding. God wants to love His people
and seeks to evoke in them a free response of love in
return. The hesed is also demanding in that God will
not be satisfied with anything less than the best efforts of His people to realize their potential and destiny. The hesed is given ethical expression in the
Decalogue or Ten Commandments. The Ten Laws stipulate
what God expects from His people in their relationship
to Him and each other. Since God extends hesed or a
faithful love to them, God expects them to love Him and
each other in a similar fashion. Likewise, The Christian experience speaks about love in terms of agape.
That is, agape is a love which is selfless and seeks only the good of the other without any hope of reward or
even being repaid. Not only is virtue its only reward,
but the ability to love in an unselfish and non-manipu-
lative way is its own reward and the highest expression
of what it means to be an authentic human being. The
principle of care places the medical professional within these two experiences. The medical professional who
accepts care as the norm of daily hospital conduct
seeks to be faithful, unselfish, and nonmanipulative in
his or her encounters with the patient and hospital
community as a whole. Care - in light of hesed and a-
gape, evoke in the medical professional a committment
to each individual patient beyond the concerns of utility, social worth, or the calculations of reward. The
medical professional who structures his or her conduct
according to care treats the patient always and in every way as a person commanding the highest respect and
dignity. Care does not ask what can the patient do,
what can the patient contribute to social life, or how
much can the patient pay for what he or she receives.
Care does not ask at all; care extends a fidelity of
concern for the best interest of each patient who comes
under my care.

The question arises: How is the principle or norm
of care applied in everyday hospital life? Care is
fundamentally an attitude, a state of being - with and
for others, a way of presenting ourselves in everyday
life. In effect, before care is a specific attitude
it is an attitude and personal committment. The attitude of and committment to care is exhibited through
caring actions. But first care is internal and then
becomes manifest in our external behavior. To be quite
specific, care is manifest in the quality of our relationship with the patient; a relationship of care is

essentially one of TRUST. Trust is the active expression of care. Why is care so closely related to trust?

One of the great pioneers in the field of understanding human behavior is Harvard psychiatrist Erik K. Erikson. Doctor Erikson in his years of research has developed eight stages in the development and maturity of the human personality. The first and most crucial stage in the process of personality development is what Doctor Erikson calls "basic trust". Basic trust involves the first years of life in which the infant forms a basic and lasting orientation towards the world. The child through contact principally with the mother (or substitute) comes to form a trustful, giving orientation towards the world, or the child because of deprivation and neglect, comes to view the world in a fearful manner. These early or first experiences are crucially important in the formation of the infant's basic orientation to life at large. The fundamental orientation of the person towards reality is rooted in these first year experiences. The child develops and grows in a mature way through the other stages (trust, autonomy, industry, initiative, identity, intimacy, generative, and integrity) only if this first stage is successfully negotiated. Without the development of basic trust the other seven stages will be severely impoverished.

We can use Doctor Erikson's insight about the importance of basic trust and apply it to the relationship between the medical professional and the patient. For without basic trust as the active element of the principle of care, the healing process is severely limited. The patient is often vulnerable as the new born child. In many ways more so. For the patient enters the hospital setting in a condition of illness and hurt. The defenses are weak and the patient is not at his or her best emotionally as well as physically. The patient enters the hospital from a position of weakness and need. The patient is quite literally at the mercy of those whom he or she encounters. The patient enters the hospital setting at a decided disadvantage. The hospital is a setting of mystery, fear, and uncertainty. The patient is preoccupied with his or her illness and the anxiety that all illness evokes. The hospital is a place in which knowledge is the most important commodity. This knowledge is highly technical in nature and vocabulary. The patient feels cut off and alienated from what is happening to him, but not necessarily because of him. Very often the patient becomes reduced

23

to a given medical procedure or markings on a chart. For example, a patient is to receive a series of x-rays. The patient encounters a world completely foreign to his or her everyday experiences. The world of the technologist is filled with machines, technical terms, and special skills. The patient experiences a certain "culture shock" in that he or she is transported from the world of everyday experience to the world of high specialization. The taken-for-granted way of acting and valuing is now set aside. In order to successfully navigate this experience the patient must trust, and the patient will trust to the extent that the medical professional exhibits care.

To conclude our discussion of care it should be remembered that the medical professional is in possession of a great deal of knowledge. The conventional wisdom assures us that "knowledge is power". However, the crucial question for the entire medical community is whether knowledge also yields virtue. The medical community must never tire of living the examined life which places high at its agenda of perennial concerns the question as to whether our knowledge is for human growth or just an end in itself. We must always ask if our growth in knowledge enables us to better serve the needs of the patient. In effect, does our growth in knowledge of a technical sort increase our sensitivity to the need for growth in the moral realm. In effect, the principle of care seeks to educate, that is liberate, the medical professional in a total way. Care demands that the medical professional be technically competent and in possession of the necessary knowledge to perform those tasks essential to the healing enterprise. Likewise, care demands that we grow as a person who exhibits prudence and sensitivity to the patient's human needs. This double educational thrust of care as technical and human competence is essential to the healing art. Without,it, we perform without committment; we encounter the patient without care; and basic trust will never be realized.

CHAPTER III

THE MEDICAL PROFESSIONAL AND THE HOSPITAL COMMUNITY

The moral life is essentially a life of being-with and being-for others. The everyday life of the medical professional is equally "people centered". Morality and medicine come together in the concern for the individual and society. It is unfortunate to think that the essentials of the medical professional are testtubes, charts, machines, and various medical routines. The fundamental entity in the everyday world of the medical professional is the individual patient who is in need of care and healing. The technical expertise of the medical profession is for the service of the patient. All of our efforts at learning and our years of study have as their goal the health and care of the patient. We can never permit ourselves to wander too far from the individual patients we seek to serve each day.

The moral life and the everyday concerns of the medical professional involve us deeply with humankind. We are reminded of our social nature and our basic dependency on others. Initially that can cause us some discomfort. In the past ten years there has been a tremendous emphasis on the self. Some writers have termed the seventies the "Me Decade". There was an overemphasis on self-improvement and self-control. In and of itself there is nothing wrong with personal development; however, such efforts should not isolate us from the concerns of others and society. Also we tend to view relationships as inhibiting our freedom. There has been a fear on the part of some to make a commitment to another person, some ideal, or a work that needs to be done. At times we want to "play it cool", "keep our options open", and "hang loose". Relationships and a personal investment of the self can evoke fear. Maybe too much will be asked of us. Maybe more than we can give will be required. However, to be a medical professional is to be part of a vital and unique community - a community dedicated to healing and care of the patient as a person. The medical professional is vital to the life of the hospital community. The contributions and the quality of our effort to hospital life are related to the depth of our self-commitment. Hospital life will not afford us the luxury of a half-hearted effort. Only our best work in accordance with professional and ethical standards are acceptable. To be part of a hospital community is to refuse to escape to an island and be isolated. The medical professional is a person who is part of a great community effort that works together with the patient to promote healing. The medical professional is involved in four basic interpersonal relationships: the self, the patient, one's peer group, and the supervisory staff. It is important to examine our relationship with each of these.

THE SELF. The fundamental relationship which effects and directs all of our interpersonal encounters is the quality of relationship we have with ourselves. Very often this is the most overlooked and disvalued of all relationships, yet, it is the most important one. We cannot relate in a mature and caring way to others if we are not able to relate in a mature and caring way to the self. Each of is in in possession of two interrelated selves: the real self (R) and the ideal self (I). Both are necessary for a mature, healthy self-concept. The R-self is the person we actually are with all of our limitations, skills, talents, and weaknesses. The R-self is the person we are without pretensions or excuses. The I-self is the self we want or hope to be. It is the self that realizes potential and eliminates human weakness. The mature self-concept seeks to balance the demands of the I-self ("you must do better") with the recognition of limitations offered by the R-self ("well, you are only human"). The mature self does not build up high levels of anxiety in an impossible attempt to obtain some ideal that cannot be reached. The I-self can place great demands on the person in a totally unrealistic way. No accomplishment is worthwhile and no effort is sufficient to satisfy the I-self. This often produces a poor self-image in which we are filled with feelings of inadequacy and worthlessness. On the other hand, we cannot give in totally to the R-self. The R-self tends to accept things the way they are and be satisfied with status-quo. However, satisfaction can easily become complacency and an excuse for growth. The I-self is necessary as the motivation for the R-self to do better because the R-self can do better, and not because the I-self demands it. In other words, the R-self and I-self are in dialogue with each other, and because they work together growth is realized. The development of a positive and mature self-image is crucial to our growth as medical professionals and human beings.

It is often true that in our work and care for others we overlook the need to extend such care to

26

ourselves. The I-self convinces us that we are more
than human and are not in need of the basic necessities
of our health: proper rest, relaxation, exercise, bal-
anced diet, and quiet time for meditation. These are
not luxuries that we give to ourself, rather, they are
the necessities we owe ourself if we are to effectively
care for the patient and interact with others in a mature way. It is easy for us out of a false sense of
duty and dedication to overlook the essentials for our
own proper health. Recently in California (1980) a new
state law was enacted by the California Medical Association which attempts to overcome the reluctance of doctors to recognize and deal with impaired colleagues.
Doctors (and we might add all medical professionals who
must learn to deal with high levels of stress) are subject to the same human limitations that effect the rest
of humanity. Medical professionals are subject to al-
coholism, drug abuse, mental illness, and the tension
that comes with the demands of career and family life.
For example, as many as ten percent of California's
30,000 practicing doctors may have drug, liquor, or
mental problems. The stress factor is highest for the
health care technician and the nursing professional,
more so even for the physician. In a study of 130 oc-
cupations conducted by the National Institute for Oc-
cupational Safety and Health the highest stress jobs
were related to direct health care. Physicians, sur-
prisingly, ranked a very low 106 out of 130, whereas,
health care para-professionals rank in the top 30. The
reason offered by research groups was that physicians
experienced less stress due to the fact they are in
control of the situation. The physician's actions can
reduce tension by the mere fact that one is doing something. The para-medical professional is often in the
same situation as the family or loved one: both can
only wait and with that waiting often comes feelings of
powerlessness and stress. The physician initiates the
action and the para-medical professional must wait for
such orders and react to them.

The normal (not to mention those days of extra-
ordinary pressure) hospital day is often filled with
hectic, demanding tasks. If we are to do what is required in a human way we need to develop the discipline
of taking time to relax and be refreshed during the
hospital day. This can be done on our breaks or lunch
hour with some quiet time alone. This will only come
with personal resolve on our part and an effort by supervisory personnel to see that such moments are taken.
The medical professional should not be made to feel

27

guilty or undedicated for such moments; in fact, these moments should be valued as a sign of maturity on the part of the professional. The need to extend care to ourselves is powerfully captured in the following words of psychiatrist Carl Jung:

Is there ever a doubt in my mind that it is virtuous for me to give alms to the beggar, to forgive him who offends me, yes, even to love my enemy in the name of Christ? No, not once does such a doubt cross my mind, certain as I am that what I have done unto the least of my brethren, I have done unto Christ.

But what if I should discover that the least of all brethren, the poorest of all beggars, the most insolvent of all offenders, yes, even the very enemy himself - that these live within me, that I myself stand in need of the arms of my own kindness, that I am to myself the enemy who is to be loved - what then?

THE PATIENT. In the development of a good self-image we are better able to relate to the patient, our colleagues, and the supervisory staff. The most obvious relationship that the health care professional forms is with the patient. In many ways the quality of the relationship that one forms with each patient will determine the effectiveness of the care offered. There are at least three basic ways to view the patient and the relationship we develop with each patient.

(A) UTILITY. In viewing the patient in a utilitarian way we ask the following: How useful, productive, or socially worthwhile is this patient? Such a perspective is not concerned with the individual dignity of each person as a human being, but the value of the individual calculated in terms of some extrinsic measure (money, social status, or contributions to society). The value of each person is defined in a rather fluid and subjective way depending on what is valued at a given time in a particular place. The weak, sick, retarded, and elderly can be viewed as a burden to society and an economic drain. When people cease to be useful to a society in some functional way it is all too easy to eliminate them on the grounds of social well-being. The Nazi experience is an enduring and tragic lesson to what happens when the value and dignity of each person is dependent upon social utility and political recognition. It is all too easy to define certain human beings as less than human.

28

(B) <u>RATIONALISM</u>. American society, and societies in general, accord a great deal of respect and rewards to individuals who exhibit high intellectual achievement. A recent development in California attests to the degree to which some prize intelligence. The sperm of certain Nobel winners has been collected and used to fertilize the eggs of selected women of high IQ's in hope of fostering future generations endowed with "Nobelintelligence". This breeding for IQ is a classic example of the belief that high intelligence yields individuals of high virtue and high intelligence will enable us to solve all our problems. However, such solutions often ignore two crucial factors: environment and the lessons of history. Intelligence is social in its development. The mind grows through interpersonal contact. The proper environment is essential for the cultivation of one's native intelligence. Also, history teaches that intelligence does not automatically insure ethical behavior. Few would doubt the intelligence of Hitler or Stalin; however, few would recommend their ethical code of conduct. There are strong currents to equate the value of the individual with one's intellectual achievements. Under stress and tension it is all too easy to become intolerant of people who don't easily understand our medical directions. Such intolerance can view the patient as stupid, hostile, or not having a genuine desire to get well. Such labeling, however, only adds to the problem and deepens the tension. What is often interpreted as lack of intelligence or a negative attitude is in reality an anxiety on the part of the patient which inhibits communication. A great deal of patience on the part of the medical professional is required.

(C) <u>PERSONALISM</u>. The moral depth of each society can be measured by the degree to which it values <u>all</u> its members regardless of their social usefulness and intellectual abilities. The medical community is measured by the same standards: the depth of its commitment to the care of each person regardless of utility, social status, intelligence, and ability to pay. The medical community is governed by the following principle: The patient is forever a person in whose debt we stand and who lays claim to our care and respect. The personalist perspective seeks to make those in the medical profession sensitive to the following factors:

1. Each person whom I encounter is <u>unique</u> and has individual talents, skills, weaknesses, and a life-story. There are no two patients who are exactly alike

29

or who are mass-produced. There is a need to be sensitive to individual differences and an appreciation of such differences.

2. There is a tremendous need to be sensitive to the sociological and situational factors in patient care. Among the sociological factors of note are: education, income level, age, and the ethnic and racial heritage of the patient. A sensitivity to these factors can help the medical professional to relate in a more understanding way to the patient. It should be remembered that illness is not only objective, but is deeply subjective and requires an interpretation on the part of the patient. Sociological factors contribute greatly to the way in which an illness or trauma is understood and coped with. In addition to sociological factors, the medical professional needs to be attentive to the context in which the patient is encountered along with the patient's family and loved ones. There are conditions and locations in the hospital which are high pressure areas, for example, the emergency room, intensive care, surgery, recovery, the psychiatric and cardiac units, along with the nurseries and maternity sections. These areas call for great sensitivity and tact in dealing with the patient and especially the family who are experiencing anxiety and concern. The loved ones of the patient often will press for some information concerning the patient. Such requests must be handled in a very understanding way. However, all such requests should be directed to the physician or the nursing staff directly responsible for that patient.

3. The hospital setting is a second home to the medical professional. Hospital life, language, and procedures are part of the medical professional's everyday world. However, what is normal to the professional is very abnormal and threatening to the patient. What the professional takes for granted very often fills the patient with anxiety. The following forms of behavior usually result from being insensitive to the feelings of the patient and can be eliminated through a professional sensitivity on our part.

A. UNNECESSARY HASTE. There is a great therapeutic value in listening to the patient and allowing him or her to talk. Talking is often a sign of anxiety and the effort to relieve such fears. We often want to silence the patient believing that such talk is useless and only delays us in doing our work. However, there are many instances in which we can do both - we can

30

converse with the patient and at the same time perform in a very professional manner what is required. Also unnecessary haste should be eliminated especially with the elderly patient who finds movement difficult and painful.

B. UNNECESSARY REMARKS. Very often we think out loud. However, such thinking can be very upsetting or embarassing to the patient. For example, if we are having a difficult time with a patient we may feel and think: what a difficult patient!; this just isn't my day; or what did I do to deserve this. We may feel this way, but we should never express aloud thes feelings. Also, there are times when the medical procedures we are attempting to do are not going well. We can't find the vein. The patient can't or won't hold his breath. The frustration we experience during such moments is not helped by vocalizing our frustration. However, innocent or justified we feel such remarks are they can humilate the patient and increase patient defensiveness.

C. EMOTIONAL DISPLAY. The medical professional as a professional must maintain control of his or her emotions at all times. Displays of anger, irritation, and frustration are a clear and disturbing signal to the patient that we have lost our effectiveness. When we act out of control the quality of care extended to the patient is severely impaired. The hospital setting is often filled with tension. The medical professional works long hours and the patient may be waiting equally long hours with the result that nerves are on edge. The medical professional through sensitivity and patience must always seek to defuse such potentially explosive situations.

D. DIAGNOSING. The patient is naturally curious about the results of tests and procedures he or she endures. After all, they have the most to gain or lose from them. Anyone who has information about the outcome is sought out by the patient. Naturally the patient thinks that the one who performed the procedure is the best qualified to interpret the findings. Therefore, the patient will often pressure the medical professional for information. Such inquiry should be viewed as natural and handled with understanding. All inquiries should be referred to the physician or someone in proper authority. There is a strong temptation not to seem ignorant or be without sufficient knowledge. Again, our ideal self is working its compulsive demands

31

to be more than what is reasonable and proper. Personal maturity and adherence to professional standards and essentials shall guide in such situations.

4. The personalist perspective is not only negative, that is, what should be avoided, but it is essentially positive. This positive thrust of the personalist approach is manifest in the following ways:

A. The personalist perspective seeks to increase the medical professional's sensitivity to the needs of the patient. The comfort and well-being of the patient is of upper-most importance. This sensitivity is often expressed in little ways such as seeing that the patient is warm, providing a pillow, gently assisting the patient, and taking a few moments to explain the procedure. All of these and many others can indicate to the patient how much we value them and our dedication to health care.

B. The greatest sensitivity is needed in dealing with the patient in certain procedures. The medical professional must always seek to protect the dignity of the patient through the proper exercise of modesty. Modesty is the proper exercise of conduct which indicates to the patient that we respect their person and dignity. Modesty is very important in dealing with the elderly patient. The exercise of modesty demands tact and maturity on the part of the medical professional. For example, in certain radiologic procedures such as mammograms and various barium studies that patient's dignity must be protected through the proper exercise of modesty and professional behavior.

C. A good part of our relationship with the patient involves our making requests of the patient (stop breathing, move a certain way, etc.). This request making should be done in a self-assured, nonthreatening manner. Such an approach evokes feelings of confidence in the patient. To be self-assured ought not to be confused with being arrogant. Our attitude can either elicit the co-operation of the patient, or we can raise the patient's anxiety and defensiveness. Also we should not by our words or actions give the patient cause to doubt us. Often we articulate our uncertainties out loud, such as, "what x-ray technique should I use?"; "I am not sure what the doctor wants me do do"; or "I am having trouble finding the vein." All of these may be true, however, it is best for all concerned if the patient does not know.

32

Finally, our request of the patient should be done in a clear, distinct, and simple manner so as to reduce confusion.

PROFESSIONAL COLLEAGUES. One of the most satisfying aspects of any profession is the valuable and lasting relationships that one is able to form. These relationships offer an invaluable source of encouragement, support, and growth through the sharing of common experiences and concerns. The fostering of professional relationships is one of the most crucial steps in the formation of a mature personality. The ability to form such relationships with professional colleagues is an indication that one is not threatened by others who have similar concerns and insights that can help us grow. The mature professional is able to cooperate with others and not fear manipulation, or be suspicious and distrustful of others. The mature professional does not operate out of a frightened sense of pseudo-independence, but seeks out his or her colleagues for their advice and experience. The mature professional cannot be a lone wolf doing one's own thing and insulated from the cooperation and criticism of the community. A true professional is eager to form close colleague relationships and welcomes criticism as a valuable asset to his or her professional performance.

Even if one does not value professional relationships because of the growth they offer, one could value them on pragmatic grounds. Namely, the vast majority of jobs and promotions are awarded on the basis of one's ability to relate with others. The professional is in the people business, and this is certainly true of the medical professional. The Carnegie Institute of Technology has determined that 85% of job success is related to personality factors and 15% is related to technical training. Harvard University in a similar study has determined that for every person who lost a job because of technical incompetence, two lost their job due to failure in dealing with others. The medical professional, in order to be successful, must develop technical competence and a mature ability to relate with others.

One of the major issues that affect relationships between colleagues is that of criticism. We need to distinguish between constructive and destructive criticism. Constructive criticism is essential to personal and professional growth. Without criticism we would never advance and we would be severely limited by our own experience and insights. However, constructive criticism is a sign of care and concern on the part of others. It is not easy to criticize; in fact, it is much easier to live with the status quo and overlook the shortcomings of others. It is a sign of respect when someone takes the time and effort to dare to criticize. The one to offer criticism is willing to suffer our anger, misunderstanding, and resentment. Our response to constructive criticism is a good indication of our own personal maturity. We can take such criticism in a negative way and view it as everyone being against us or no one appreciating our efforts. We can give in to self-pity. Or we can grow and be appreciative of the efforts of others to correct our faults and improve our professional behavior. The mature professional who has enough ego-strength and a good self-image welcomes criticism and even seeks it out. He or she knows that in so doing the quality of care extended to the patient is greatly improved.

Not all criticism is constructive however. There are instances when destructive criticism is advanced. Such criticism is often motivated by the "green-eyed monster" we call jealousy. Destructive criticism is offered from one who is basically insecure and feels that the only way he or she can feel adequate is by bringing others down. Just the opposite often occurs. This game of "draw down the other to my level" is quickly uncovered and one who plays such a game often loses the respect of one's colleagues and the support of the professional community. There are many motives or reasons why we criticize others. Destructive criticism can be motivated by jealousy, but also because we see our own faults and limitations in others. Therefore, if we can condemn them in others, psychologically it gives us a feeling of superiority and relieves us of guilt. Also, destructive criticism is a sign of immaturity on our part along with a poor self-image. Destructive criticism is usually a projection of criticism offered by the Ideal-Self to the Real-Self which the individual cannot handle. Therefore this criticism is projected on to others in an attempt to relieve anxiety. Once again criticism is essential to growth and is essential to our professional development. However, all criticism should be done in the right place, at the right time, and by the appropriate person.

To be a professional is to be part of a community. The medical professional is involved in a daily contact with one's professional community or colleagues. This intimate and intense contact can cause stress insensitivity. This is especially true in terms of one's speech habits. The most destructive element of community and professional life along with jealousy is that of gossip. Man is the language animal. We use words to make sense of our everyday world and experience. The richer our vocabulary the more zestful our experience of life. The pattern of our everyday speech reveals a great deal about us as a person and a professional. Gossip is a good indicator of personal immaturity and lack of professional commitment to our colleagues. Gossip is the disrespectful and obscene misuse of language. Gossip reveals to others who and what we really are. The enticing element in gossip is its supposedly secret nature. We are priviliged to know what others do not. We have the "inside" information. We are blessed with a superior knowledge that others do not have. We often feel honored when one shares gossip with us, especially about another. However, if we remember that if one speaks to us <u>about another</u> in time that same person will speak to another <u>about us</u>. Gossip is the opposite of the virtue prudence and the professional standard of confidentiality. Prudence is the exercise of the practical intelligence which is evidenced through good judgment. This good judgment is called for in knowing when to keep silent and when to speak. The medical professional is in the priviliged position of knowing a good deal about the patient and one's colleagues and staff. The way in which we manage such information goes a long way in determining the quality of colleague relationships and personal maturity. (More will be said about confidentiality in the next chapter (MEDICO-LEGAL RESPONSIBILITIES.)

<u>AUTHORITY FIGURES</u>. Ours is not a time which finds authority easy to obey or exercise. We have come to define freedom as the doing of one's own thing and the lack of external controls. In effect, freedom has been associated with a whimsical subjectivism and an overall negativism. However, we cannot be content to be free <u>from</u> this or that restraint; we must ask what we are free <u>for</u>. Also the mature exercise of freedom requires that we recognize all true freedom has its limits. Freedom only becomes meaningful when it is applied in the real world. In the application of freedom through choice we always give up and accept some limit on ourselves. Genuine freedom demands self-limitation. For example, in choosing to become a medical professional one freely decides not to be an elementary school teacher or a mechanical engineer. To be

mature and properly exercise freedom we must limit ourselves to a set of given circumstances and options. Freedom becomes the being free for this or that course of action which determines the kind of person we become. In effect, freedom demands discipline for its proper exercise and a clear vision of goals in the decisions we make. Such freedom is a far cry from the subjective do what you want concept that is so popular today.

Authority is essential in the proper functioning of a hospital and to insure quality care for the patient. There is a need for authority and a chain of responsibility in the working of any organization, and most especially a hospital. For those of us who are in positions of authority and responsibility this is an awesome trust and sacred responsibility. The mature exercise of authority means that one welcomes criticisms and questions from subordinates done in good faith and the search for truth. The mature supervisor does not want docile and immature obedience which is often a mask for resentment on the part of those under our authority. The mature supervisor seeks to foster a maturity in others so they can make decisions and accept responsibility. Contrary to popular opinion, the worst thing that can be said about a leader or person of authority is that the community can't get along without them. The mature leader does not want to be indispensable. Often the desire to make oneself indispensable results from insecurity and weak ego-strength. The greatest exercise of our authority is that we care and trust others to take control and responsibility for their lives. Conflicts are natural and to be expected when highly motivated people work so closely together in situations of stress. However, there is nothing to be gained by raw displays of power or blind ambition that make one insensitive to the dignity of others. Authority is most necessary and appreciated when it is exercised in moments of tension in a way that respects the worth of each person. Through the exercise of such authority one becomes a person not only in authority (a position or role), but also of authority (a recognition on the part of others that one has a moral right to exercise the authority related to one's role).

Regardless of one's position and authority few if any of us are free from accountability. Not only do we possess authority but we are also under authority. There is a very close relationship between the way in which one exercises authority and acts while under authority. One cannot demand obedience on the part of others all the while resenting and challenging the legitimate authority of others. The para-medical professional is subject to authority in many forms: from physicians, supervisors, teachers, and one's colleagues in positions of greater seniority. Our relationship to those in authority will go a long way in determining our professional and personal growth. Above all, one must avoid extremes, that is, a mindless, slavish obedience which really masks our fear of authority, and one must avoid a childish rebellion which shows a complete lack of discipline. The mature response to authority involves one in the need to be respectful, courteous, and understanding while at the same time exercising proper self-respect and a questioning attitude. One is neither a slave or a rebel, but a mature person and professional seeking to care for the patient in the best possible way.

In bringing this section and chapter to a close, a few words should be said about one's relationship to the institution or physician under whom one is working. The medical professional owes a debt of gratitude to the hospital or school in which they received their training. This gratitude is expressed in various ways: loyalty to one's obligations and duties, respect for persons and positions in authority, honesty in dealing with oneself and others especially with regard to professional standards, and finally, a mature openness to criticism. To be a medical professional is to be involved with human beings on many levels. The quality of patient care can only be improved to the extent that the entire hospital community works together in a professional manner to achieve that goal.

CHAPTER IV

MEDICO-LEGAL RESPONSIBILITIES
OF THE MEDICAL PROFESSIONAL

The attitude of many today toward the law is one of negativity and even open hostility. The law is often viewed as an unnecessary limitation on our freedom. The contemporary mind often associates obedience to the law with nothing more than stale duty or mindless conformism. The Watergate episode along with many recent political scandals have disillusioned many to the function of law in society and the legal and political professions in general. Laws often seem to interfere with the smooth operation of our daily life. Laws are sometimes viewed as being for the advantage of the powerful to the detriment of the poor or powerless. Laws in the area of morality have fallen into decay and are often viewed as legalisms or prejudices from a by-gone era. Moral laws have come to be viewed by some as an attempt on the part of elites in society to legitimate their privileges and control.

However, in our more thoughtful moments we realize how essential law is to society and the quality of life within society. Without law life would be in the words of the philosopher Thomas Hobbes, "short, cruel, and brutish". Without law life would be reduced to survival of the fittest based on raw displays of power. The absence of law is not freedom but chaos. The abuses of law are all too evident and real. No one really disputes this. However, it should be remembered that the abuse of something is not a sufficient argument against its proper use. The law, when properly formulated, is the result of society's reflection on experience and challenges it faces. Law in its better moments is the result of reasoned consideration by society in seeking to promote order, justice, and the common good. Contemporary life is characterized by bigness and the need for law is essential to secure the rights of all citizens. Laws are far from perfect, mainly because they are formulated by far from perfect human societies. However, when one considers the alternative, there is really no alternative.

The law permeates the whole of society and includes the practice of medicine in all its forms. In fact, the law has exerted tremendous influence in the field of health care in recent years, for example,

national health insurance, the allocation of scarce resources through tax allocation for research, the formation of guidelines in various bio-medical research pro-
jects such as DNA studies, and the legislative action
of various states in forming guidelines to determine
when a person can be legally declared dead. Every profession in a society seeks recognition for the work it
does and the knowledge its members possess. In other
words, to be a professional is to stake a claim for social recognition and status. With all status claims
come social responsibilities and duties to one's profession and the society at large. The claims of a society in protecting the interest of all citizens and
insuring the quality of professional behavior is expressed through law and guidelines. The medical profession is one of the most powerful and crucial to the
quality of life in a modern society. Therefore, it
seems only natural that the presence of the law should
be an integral part of the medical establishment. It
becomes increasingly necessary for medical professionals to be aware of how the law effects them and what
are the legal responsibilities of the various professions.

In our discussion of the legal aspects that effect
the medical profession, two points must be kept in
mind: first, our remarks are limited to the para-medical professionals, most especially those who work in
the various medical technical fields such as x-ray and
the various laboratory professionals. Secondly, in
discussing the law it is easy to fall into a minimalis-
tic approach to one's work. The law sets limits, often in negative terms, as to what is to be avoided in
caring for the patient. The guidelines and standards
of the medical professions often go beyond the basic
requirements of the law. The true professional seeks
to obey the law, but is never satisfied with only ful-
filling the basics. Having offered these two qualifi-
ers, we now turn our attention to a discussion of some
of the basic legal realities as related to medicine.
We will also discuss some practical guidelines for proper patient care in order to avoid legal negligence.
Finally, we will discuss the important aspect of confidentiality in relationship to the patient and in dealing with other health care professionals.

The para-medical professional is viewed in the
eyes of the law as an _employee_. That is, the para-medical professional is under the direct supervision of a
physician. Also, the para-medical professional is an

employee since he or she renders a service. However, to say that the para-medical professional is under the supervision of a physician does not mean that the para-medical professional is free from all legal responsibilities for his or her actions. The para-medical professional is capable of committing what in legal terminology is called a tort. A tort is an act for which one is held legally responsible. The basis for determining torts is the criteria of the reasonable person acting according to proper standards of medical practice and the anticipation of reasonable consequences for a given action. In other words, the basic issue of torts is as follows: if an injury or death occurs through one's action or failure to act, the law wants to know would the reasonable person in the same capacity and circumstances have acted in a similar way. Let us take an example from the field of radiologic technology. The technologist is ordered by the physician to inject the patient with the radiologic media for an IVP. The physician then leaves to tend to another patient. The technologist obeys the physician, injects the patient; however, the patient is allergic, goes into cardiac arrest and dies. The radiologic technologist is liable for having exceeded his or her sphere of competence and responsibility. The radiologic technologist is not permitted to inject a patient with radiologic media regardless of the orders by the physician. The standard medical practice calls for the radiologic technologist to refrain from injections and, in addition, the reasonable person should have foreseen the possibility that the patient may react adversely to the media. In the above example the standards of accepted medical practice were violated along with a failure to anticipate reasonable consequences.

The fact that the para-medical professional can commit torts does not mean that the supervisor or physician escapes responsibility. The law recognized what it calls the tort of respondent superior ("let the master respond or answer"). This concept states that the employer, physician, hospital, or state agency is responsible or liable for torts committed by an employee in the course of one's professional behavior. Liability runs both ways - employee and employer. The rationale for such a rule has deep roots in Anglo-Saxon law which invested the power of control over one's employee in the master or head of the factory or manor. This may strike us today as paternalistic or out of date; however, the high rate of insurance charged to employers and companies attest to the everyday reality of such a legal concept. The employer who hires a person for a task is also making a statement about the trustworthiness and reliability of the employee. The employer, in contracting a given individual, is at the same time accepting responsibility for how this individual will behave in the carrying out of one's duties related to the job. To be an employer is to have power; it is also a call to responsibility and the need to exercise prudence in the selection of those who come into our employ. The exercise of such prudence in hiring by supervisory staff and physicians is most essential in the field of health care. Not only must the prospective employee be technically competent, but he or she should be a person of character and moral sensitivity.

The vast majority of legislation involving medical personnel and the patient center around offenses of negligence. It is often not so much what we do as what we fail to do that causes injury to the patient and compromises the quality of patient care. Negligence can be defined in the following way: negligence is the failure to exercise the care which a person of ordinary prudence and following accepted standards of medical practice would use under the same or similar circumstances. Negligence is the failure to observe reasonable care in the exercise of one's duties. Negligence often results from at least four attitudes deficiences: carelessness, inattention, ignorance, and confusion. Carelessness is the failure to carry out our procedures and instructions in a professional and competent way. One does not pay significant attention to detail which compromises patient care. Inattention is the failure to concentrate in the carrying out of one's duties in relation to the patient and that which affects the patient (equipment, condition of the examination room, I-V medication, etc.). Ignorance is the failure on the part of the medical professional to keep abreast of standard technical practices. The need to be current with one's field is not merely a technical requirement, but is also an ethical one. The medical professional has a moral responsibility to provide the best care possible to each patient under his or her care. Confusion is often the result of lack of preparation by the medical professional for a given procedure. If one fails to be properly prepared and be prepared for the unexpected, stress is increased and accidents occur. Confusion due to lack of preparation reduces efficiency and limits the quality of patient care. These attitude deficiencies can be overcome by a dedication and self-discipline which accentuates a careful attention to detail, the effort to keep well-informed about one's field, and a determination to be prepared for both the routine and unexpected in the carrying out of one's duties.

The failure to exercise proper care, follow standard medical practice, and anticipate reasonable consequences often results in accidents. The following is a list, by no means exhaustive, of some of the more obvious and necessary situations in which professional alertness and competence are essential.

1. __The emergency or accident room.__ One must be sensitive to the condition of the patient and the obvious concern of family members and loved ones. The emergency room is a high stress area in which preparation, speed, and professional competence are of the utmost necessity. The need for the medical professional to be in control of his or her self is essential and this comes with the knowledge that one is competent in one's field.

2. __Psychiatric patient.__ The medical professional needs to exercise the greatest prudence and alertness in carrying out one's various procedures. The psychiatric attendant should always be close at hand and encouraged to assist in whatever way possible to insure proper care and a safe examination for all concerned. The medical professional can be of great assistance to the psychiatric staff if he or she reports any rapid change in behavior or mood. There is a need to be calm and reduce as much as possible tension and stress in a given procedure. This can often be accomplished by explaining, if possible, what is going to take place. If the patient knows ahead of time what will take place this can greatly reduce anxiety.

3. __Prisoners and the Intoxicated.__ From time to time the para-medical professional is called upon to care for those who are at odds with society. However, the highest professional standards and non-judgmental attitudes must be exercised. The medical professional is not called upon to pass judgment upon those held in prisons or those arrested who are brought to the hospital for treatment. Those who are at odds with the law still command our respect and care. The medical professional should be prepared to work quickly and exercise extreme caution in caring for the patient. Whenever possible, the appropriate legal authorities should be present during the various procedures.

4. <u>Maternity patients and Infant care</u>. The expectant mother, the new-born, or pre-mature baby pose special problems for the radiologic technologist. The need to practice proper radiation protection techniques is of the utmost importance. The general public has been hearing a great deal about the dangers of x-ray exposure. This fear may be or seem to be groundless to the radiologic technologist; however, as a professional one should exercise the utmost care and try to educate the public about x-ray technology. Part of this education can be provided by our professional behavior and standards of proper care. X-ray exposure should be kept to a minimum especially to the expectant mother and the new or pre-mature born baby. In addition, when one is doing portable x-rays or x-rays in populated areas (recovery and surgery) proper protection should be offered to those in the area. One should announce that an x-ray is about to be taken. Finally, many maternity patients need x-ray procedures which call for <u>erect</u> procedures. One needs to be sure the patient is properly secured to the table and the foot device for erect procedures are properly fastened. On many erect procedures there is a tendency for the patient to faint or experience disequilibrium. This often results from blood rapidly leaving the brain and settling in the lower part of the body. Such fainting or disequilibrium can be reduced by bringing the table slowly from the supine to the erect position. All the while try to reassure the patient and inquire about her feelings. The same is true for all erect procedures that call for moving the patient from the supine to erect position.

In addition to these various situations and conditions of the patient, accidents can be avoided by exercising reasonable judgment in terms of having one's work area clean and unencumbered. This can reduce the possibility of the patient falling over a misplaced piece of equipment or slipping on a wet floor. In addition, great care should be exercised in doing procedures which call for the patient to remove dressings or bandages. The elderly patient often suffers from arthritis. Movement is painful and the need for patience is fundamental. Also, many procedures call for the transfer of a patient from a stretcher to an examination or x-ray table. Great caution should be exercised and the best way to exercise such caution is to have sufficient help in assisting the patient.

In our discussion about negligence, it must be emphasized that one is not being asked to practice

"defensive health care". Good medical practice, grounded in accepted professional standards, and guided by
the reasonable exercise of one's judgment, calls the
medical professional to <u>actively</u> promote the good of
the patient. The mature medical professional does not
seek to live by the strict letter of the law. He or
she realizes that the law is a statement by society of
what it expects minimally from its members. However,
the true health care professional seeks constantly to
upgrade his or her professional standards and the quality of care administered to the patient. No one can
foresee everything that will happen. Everyone has
their limits. However, this does not excuse one from
the proper exercise of good judgment and the need to
be prepared for each procedure. To be prepared for and
sensitive to consequences, in addition to being alert
for the unexpected, means one can provide care to the
patient of the highest quality. Before proceeding to
our next chapter we need to say a brief, but necessary,
word about confidentiality.

    Confidentiality is the exercise of prudence (good
judgment) in relation to one's speaking habits. Confidentiality is the mature ability to know when to
speak and be silent and with whom one should and should
not speak. Confidentiality is fundamental to social
life and the quality of interpersonal relationships.
Each of us as human beings require opportunities to express our inner feelings and thoughts to another without fear of having them "shouted from the rooftop".
All of us need to have at least one person we can speak
to with confidence knowing that no matter what we say
or feel we will be understood and accepted. Even if we
have done wrong, society recognizes certain privileged
persons and relationships with whom one can bare one's
soul without fear of self-incrimination: priest-peni-
tent, lawyer-client, husband-wife, and to a lesser degree, physician-patient. Not only is confidentiality
essential to social and interpersonal life, it is a
time-honored principle of proper medical practice. In
fact, we can return to the Hippocratic Oath itself:
"Whatever...I see or hear...which ought no to be
spoken abroad, I will not divulge". The medical tradition upholding confidentiality is much deeper than mere
social etiquette or being good-mannered. Confidentiality lies at the heart of the medical professional-pa-
tient relationship. It is essential for proper care
and the formation of trust. Confidentiality demands
one respect the right to privacy of the patient and
one's colleagues in terms of medical treatment and

records.

The principle of confidentiality is not an absolute value in proper medical care and conduct. There are circumstances in which the medical professional is called upon to make known to the proper authorities certain situations and conditions which threaten the common good. These are situations in which to keep silent would be an act of irresponsibility and this could be the cause of great harm. For example, one is required to notify the proper authorities in instances of suspected child abuse, gun shot wounds, and those who have contracted communicable diseases that would endanger the health of the population at large. Other instances also come to mind, such as the drug addict who uses methadone not for his own habit, but uses it for resale in order to buy heroin. The medical professional would be required to notify proper officials. There are many more examples, however, the point we are attempting to make is simply this: in the vast majority of cases, under normal circumstances, the right to privacy must be protected through the proper exercise of confidentiality. Only under the most pressing of circumstances is one obliged to reveal what one comes to know in the course of one's medical duties.

In bringing our remarks on confidentiality to a close, as well as this chapter, a few general guidelines about confidentiality may prove helpful.

1. The prudent exercise of confidentiality calls for the medical professional to safeguard the privacy of the patient by refusing to release information without the proper authorization. All inquiries about the treatment and condition of a given patient should be referred to the proper medical authorities.

2. Confidentiality calls for the medical professional to respect the privacy of all conversations. One should not repeat things heard between a patient and his or her family or loved ones. Often the patient will speak to a friend or relative under the assumption that what is said is privileged information. The medical professional should treat all such conversation as just that - privileged information.

3. When one is in doubt as how to handle a request for information or whether to make known what one hears in the course of an examination or procedure, the medical professional should always consult one's

supervisor or the physician in charge. This is not a
sign of immaturity; quite the contrary, it is the mark
of one who knows his or her limits and areas of responsibility. The seeking of such advice about confidentiality points out the importance of developing good
professional relationships with one's superiors.

4. Not only must one respect the conversations
between patient and loved ones, but also the medical
professional must respect the conversations between
physicians and physicians and other medical professionals. Such conversations are privileged information and
should be so treated. Many times a physician will think
out loud about possible courses of action in a given
situation. He or she may do so in order to receive
feedback from colleagues. One should respect such a
process and not divulge what was said. Sometimes physicians may differ professionally as to an appropriate
course of action or treatment of a patient. Such differences should be kept to oneself in order not to em-
barass the physicians. Also, one will soon be labeled
as trustworthy or unreliable by how one conducts oneself in such situations. It is a sign of maturity and
professional competence when one can exercise proper
prudence and self-discipline with regard to the conversations one hears.

5. The proper exercise of confidentiality forbids
one from releasing or making a diagnosis. Diagnosis is
the responsibility of the patient's physician. With
sensitivity and understanding, all inquiries about the
patient's condition should be directed to the physician.
Sometimes a patient may be involved in legal matters of
a criminal and/or civil nature. One should be very
careful in speaking about a patient's condition or
treatment. No matter how authoritative one appears or
sounds, without the proper consent of the proper medical authorities and family members no information
should be offered.

6. Finally, in our previous chapter we spoke a-
bout the destructiveness of gossip. There is often a
rationalization process which tends to paint gossip as
nothing more than the trivial exchange of news. However, for the medical professional such a rationalization in light of confidentiality cannot be tolerated.
The medical professional is privileged to know a great
deal of intimate facts about a patient and one's fellow
professionals. The degree to which one goes in honoring confidentiality is a good indicator of one's

maturity and professional commitment.

This chapter has been an attempt to highlight the need for law and how the law relates to the medical profession. We attempted to indicate as well that the law is society's statement of what is minimally required of its members as they interact on a daily basis. However, one cannot merely be satisfied to obey the letter of the law while ignoring its spirit, that is, the enhancement of the quality of life, protection of individual rights, and the securing of a more just society. In our final chapter we will focus on the medical professional as a moral agent who practices the art of healing which has as its end the healing of those who are sick and in need of care.

CHAPTER V

THE MEDICAL PROFESSIONAL AS MORAL AGENT

Society rewards and honors those members who attain certain forms of knowledge and practice various skills. Such rewards and status are society's way of encouraging and recognizing the need for a knowledgeable and skillful citizenry. In a society as technologically dependent and advanced as ours, rewards will increase in the years to come. However, society also demands a great deal from those who are in possession of such technological skills. The expectations of a society towards its elite and skillful members are given expression in legal codes as was discussed in the previous chapter. In addition to the expectation of society, many professional and technological organizations have formulated codes of ethics and professional standards of practice. These codes are often expectations beyond the minimum of the law and express a desire for professionals to maintain a high level of craftsmenship. Many professions require its members to take an oath or promise to uphold the standards and ideals of the profession. The most obvious example is the Hippocratic Oath administered to physicians. At the end of this book is a list of some of the codes of ethics and professional codes of practice required of various medical personnel.

The taking of oaths and promises have been looked upon in recent times with suspicion and skepticism. Viet-Nam, Watergate, and daily political scandals have greatly undermined the confidence of people in those in authority. This loss of confidence and believability has not been confined to the political arena. All forms of authority have been viewed with suspicion from the physician to the policeman on the beat, the priest, and the medical para-professional. There is a tendency to believe that those in authority are seeking their own advantage and do not care about the public good. Authority is often viewed as an obstacle to one's freedom and self-expression. The decade of the '60's has come and gone, but its outlook about authority has lingered on. The attitudes of suspicion, skepticism, and distrust on the part of so many make the everyday world of the professional more demanding. This is not all bad. The public is more conscious of its rights and more demanding of the services it receives. Such a critical public can provide incentive for each profession to maintain its high standards and constantly seek to upgrade the service it renders. The medical profession has come under a great deal of questioning in recent times. The high cost of medical care as well as the attitude expressed by some that the medical professional is only interested in making money have strained the traditional high esteem afforded the men and women in white. More and more the citizenry is coming to view medicine as a consumer product that one can pick and choose. In addition, this consumer approach to medicine has made the patient more militant in demanding a high quality of care as well as a guarantee to the outcome. The staggering rise in the number of medical malpractice suits is clear evidence of the consumer approach to medical care. The present situation offers the medical community a necessary and important opportunity to reexamine the goals of health care and the standards expected of those who claim to be members in good standing of the medical community.

What is the end or goal of the medical art? The end of medicine, that towards which the art-science of medicine aims, is the healing of the whole person and in the process witnessing to the primary value of human life. Medicine does not strive to repair bodies, but is concerned about the patient as a whole person: mind, body, soul, and spirit. The concept of man has been so fractured and compartmentalized in recent times. Each academic discipline offers a partial view of man and, at times unfortunately, tries to present this highly selective view as the whole of what man is. Medicine must resist this violence and view man as a unique, unified entity. Man is more than the sum of his or her parts. Man cannot be reduced to this or that fact or cause. Man can only begin to be understood when he is considered as a unified entity. In addition, the art-science of medicine is an eloquent testimony to the primary value and dignity of human life. The men and women who spend long years of study, discipline, and sacrifice do so beyond the crass rewards of status and money. The overwhelming majority do so out of a humanitarian love and concern for one's fellow and one's society. The standards of medical practice and the moral values articulated by the medical community must witness in a clear and distinct way to the value of each person. Various codes of ethics and professional standards are crucially important safeguards against those who would corrupt the fundamental aim and values of medicine for their own selfish ends. The various codes and values serve as a testament to the intrinsic worth of each person and the belief that a patient must never be turned into an object or thing for the sake of some other value no matter how noble the cause. No patient can be forced against his or her will to be part of an experiment no matter how promising or beneficial the results. To do so would run counter to the best traditions of Western philosophy, religion, and medical practice.

The need to reaffirm the goal of the medical art-science as healing for wholeness and the affirmation of the life as a primary value is of great importance today. Medicine has in recent years been struggling more and more with its tradition in terms of the goal of medicine and its relationship to the value of life. The questions of abortion, euthanasia, and human experimentation, not to mention the complex questions of death and dying, transplantation, and the issues facing the new biology, cause many to wonder and experience confusion as to where medicine and its practioners stand. The medical community, from the nurse's aide and orderly, to the technologist, to the chief-of-staff must help to develop a clear and distinct understanding of what medicine is about and how the value of each life fits into the medical picture of reality. In other words, each medical professional is called upon to contribute, question, and formulate ideas and ideals for the codes and standards that are and will be articulated for the medical community. Medicine is not the art-science of an elite few, but is a community venture in which all its members, together with the patients, help to express what is best and good in medical care. The democratization of guidelines for moral and professional behavior is a crucial step in safeguarding the individual medical professional and helping to build a more humane and just society. The stakes are too high to allow others to formulate one's ethics. To be a medical professional today is an exciting and challenging task. The medical community is at the leading edge of tomorrow and offers a real sign of hope for a more caring new day. Only a loss of nerve or apathy will turn that new day into a long night of darkness and retardation. The medical community is given the opportunity to pass on to a new generation of professionals not only a legacy of impressive technological advances, but equally important, an impressive legacy of ethical insights and wisdom to serve as a guide for the future.

The initial steps in this process of developing

moral values and standards of professional behavior is
to ask if the medical community can be satisfied with
various codes of practice, or is something more required? Perhaps instead of speaking about codes we
viewed all aspects of medical practice in the language
of covenant-relationship. Naturally we need to ask why
eliminate the word code, and secondly, just what do we
mean by the concept of covenant-relationship? A code
is a formal statement of the minimum standards of acceptable behavior and values. Codes are formal (legal
and medical profession) and informal (dress), individual and social. Codes are often related to habit, that
is, the performance of an act in a set way or method.
There is little room for creativity and imagination.
Codes can often be used as substitutes for thinking
and responding to novel situations. At its worst, a
code can lead to mindless and unreflective performance
of one's art. In effect, one's art ceases to be an
art and becomes a sterile technique. In addition,
codes can often slip into a style which is nothing more
than the correct external performance of a given technique. Ethics defined only in terms of a code too often becomes mere etiquette or aesthetics, that is, behavior which is attractive or defined as appealing.

To understand medical ethics only in terms of a
code has a serious drawback. Various medical codes often stress the importance of technical competence, however they remain silent on the issue of moral and ethical sensitivity. The moral self is often subordinated
to the technical self. Such codes clearly define what
is expected of the medical professional as he or she
practices the various medical arts. Few codes mention
any positive attitudes which should be developed by the
medical professional in relating to the patient. Medical codes which accentuate the technical self tend to
keep the medical professional at a so-called "safe distance" from the patient. One is often cautioned not to
become involved with the person in a personal way.
Codes can be used to insulate the professional from em-
pathy with the patient. A strong case can be made for
professional distance. The medical professional would
soon be emotionally "burned out" if he or she got too
involved with each patient. Ideally it would be nice
to be able to enter into the world of the patient and
share their struggles and hopes in a deep way. However, the medical professional is a human being who has
limits and needs to respect those limits. There is a
prudent need to develop a professional objectivity or
distance from the everyday world of the hospital. This

distance is essential for psychological well-being.
In this regard the various codes have much to contribute. However, such professional danger must never be
allowed to slip into professional indifference and a-
pathy. Distance is necessary so that proper medical
care can be administered to the patient; in effect, the
motivation is one of care for the patient. With apathy,
by contract, care for the patient is not a concern at
all. Apathy is an inability to feel or respond to human needs or suffering. One goes through the motions
of being a medical professional, but in reality there
is an absence of inner feeling and commitment. At
times it is very easy to confuse professional distance
with job apathy and alienation. Recent studies and
trends in medicine are convincing many that the need to
be with the patient in a human, caring way is essential
to recovery, patient confidence, and proper health
maintenance. This new trend in medical care is usually
termed holistic medicine. The holistic approach understands the end or goal of medicine to be the health of
the patient. And health is viewed as the person seeking wholeness in mind, body and spirit. Sickness is a
description of the person's well-being. Sickness frag-
ments the person. Medical care in the service of
wholeness seeks to restore the inner balance and harmony of the patient. The medical professional is not
satisfied with bodily well-being alone, but strives for
the integration and harmony of the whole person.

The medical professional does not live by codes
alone, but lives as a moral agent who applies one's art
through covenant-relationships. The basis of a covenant-relationship is the viewing of the medical professional and the patient as partners in pursuit of health.
The medical professional seeks to draw the patient into
a more active role in the healing process. The medical
professional allows and encourages the patient to tell
his or her life story and the meaning one gives to one's
illness or injury. The patient is encouraged to take
an active, responsible part in the treatment of his or
her own condition. Such an approach seeks to involve
the patient and give him or her a stake in the outcome.
This reduces the attitude of paternalism on the part of
the medical professional and challenges the patient to
act maturely toward his or her treatment. Unlike a
code, the covenant-relationship is open-ended, flexible, and is constantly sensitive to the needs of the
individual patient. The covenant-relationship cannot
be confined to legalistic do's and don'ts. But in af-
firming the dignity and worth of each patient, such

relationships always seek to do the most caring thing
for the patient in the given situation or case. The
medical professional who structures his or her everyday
in the hospital on the principle of care seeks to foster a "cannon of loyality" with the patient. This "ca-
non of loyality" or fidelity to the care of the individual patient is essential in building trust and promo-
ting healing.

In addition to covenant-relationships fostering
trust, loyalty, and care, they also remind the medical professional that he or she is in debt to the community as a whole. The medical professional owes a
debt of gratitude to so many, certainly to one's society which has set aside resources for training medical
professionals. One owes a debt to one's teachers and
family for their knowledge, support, and friendship
during and after one's formal schooling. Above all,
the medical professional owes a debt to each patient
that he or she has encountered. The realization of the
debt we owe to the patient is easy to forget with the
number of procedures one performs. This is especially
true in a teaching hospital which is often funded by
the state through tax supported funds. The poorest of
the poor as well as the richest are the one's to whom
the medical professional owes a debt of gratitude.
Naturally the question arises how is one to aprroxi-
mately express such gratitude?

In a real way no one can ever repay for the privilege of receiving an education or the gift of training
in a highly specialized field such as the modern health
professions. The closest one can come is to renew
oneself each day to provide maximum care for the patient as a person. Gratitude is expressed by a constant desire to grow in knowledge, especially beyond
the formal requirements for licensing or various registry qualifications. Some are even called to the privileged position of teaching in a formal way in helping
to train and educate future medical professionals. The
seriousness and dedication with which a teaching as-
signment is carried out goes a long way in giving to
others what one has received. However, all medical
professionals are given the opportunity to teach others by their conduct and values. Informal teaching is
in many instances the most effective way to form attitudes and habits toward proper patient care. In saying
that one can show gratitude through continuing education, dedication to professional and ethical principles, and sharing one's knowledge through teaching does

not imply that one "pays one's own way". Education and training are part of the giftedness of social and personal life. One cannot pay for it; one can only accept it in gratitude and share the gift with others.

Let us bring this chapter and inquiry to a close with the following reflection: to be a medical professional dedicated to the well-being of the patient as a person through the application of the principle of care is to assume a way of being-in-the-world. The medical professional is in-the-world-with-and-for-others in their moments of suffering and sickness. This being-with and being-for others identifies the health care professional as a person dedicated to healing. The medical professional, as one dedicated to healing, comes to view as essential to his or her self-identity this healing aspect. Healing and caring for the patient become enduring aspects of one's personal identity and everyday existence.

In saying that we bring our inquiry to an end is a bit misleading. In many ways, it is just beginning. No book or essay can cover the whole of a topic as rich and important as ethics for the health care professional. The most important contributions to our inquiry are yet to be made, and they will be made by the students, professionals, teachers, and patients now and in the future. The great hope and aim of this essay has been to provide a basic guide or point of focus for ethical and professional reflection on the quality of education and patient care that is being offered in our hospitals. Everyone will not agree with the conclusions and principles advanced in this text. In a pluralistic society this is to be expected. However, conformity is not the aim, but thinking is. The everyday experience of those who read this essay will provide the necessary enrichment and correction for its deficiences and short-sightedness. Finally, no book in ethics can make one a better health care professional or a more caring human being. Ethics is an enabling art which allows the expression of what is best in each of us. Ethics is a practical art which allows one to be sensitive to the moral dimensions of human behavior. In effect, it is not so much that ethics fails us, rather, it is we who fail ethics by indifference to our fellows. The medical art in all its forms is essentially related to the art of ethical inquiry. Both seek the growth and health of the individual and the betterment of the quality of life in general. We are living in demanding and exciting times. Nowhere is the adventure of life more intense than in the medical professions. Ethics seeks to give the medical professional guidance for today and hope for tomorrow.

Questions for Review and Discussion

1. What is ethics?

2. Briefly explain the three (3) traditional systems of doing ethics.

3. What is a norm? Explain briefly the three traditional norms of morality.

4. Why should a medical professional study ethics?

5. Explain the connection between ethics and medicine.

6. What is the principle of care and how does it relate to the everyday world of the health care professional?

7. For the Greeks knowledge is virtue. Today knowledge is more related to power. How is medical technology both virtue and power? What does this virtue-power relationship mean for the medical professional's relationship to the patient?

8. Explain the following legal aspects of medical care: tort, tort of respondent superior, the reasonable person criteria, negligence.

9. Why is confidentiality essential to the proper exercise of medical practice? Discuss some guidelines concerning confidentiality.

10. Are there ever any cases in which one is required to make known the condition of a patient without the patient's consent? Explain.

11. Explain the following: code and covenant-relationship.

12. How does one go about developing the proper balance between caring for the patient and maintaining a professional distance?

13. Why is the development of professional relationships so important for the medical professional?

14. Review your profession's code of ethics. What are its strong points? How would you improve the code?

15. Interview various patients for their view as to
    what they consider to be good medical practice.
    Did their responses surprise you? How so?

AMERICAN NURSES' ASSOCIATION
THE CODE FOR NURSES (1968)

1. The nurse provides services with respect for the dignity of man, unrestricted by considerations of nationality, race, creed, color, or status.

2. The nurse safeguards the individual's right to privacy by judiciously protecting information of a confidential nature, sharing only that information relevant to his care.

3. The nurse maintains individual competence in nursing practice, recognizing and accepting responsibility for individual actions and judgments.

4. The nurse acts to safeguard the patient when his care and safety are affected by incompetent, unethical, or illegal conduct of any person.

5. The nurse uses individual competence as a criterion in accepting delegated responsibilities and assigning nursing activities to others.

6. The nurse participates in research activities when assured that the rights of individual subjects are protected.

7. The nurse participates in the efforts of the profession to define and upgrade.

INTERNATIONAL COUNCIL OF NURSES
1973 CODE FOR NURSES
ETHICAL CONCEPTS APPLIED TO NURSING

The fundamental responsibility of the nurse is fourfold: to promote health, to prevent illness, to restore health and to alleviate suffering.

The need for nursing is universal. Inherent in nursing is respect for life, dignity and rights of man. It is unrestricted by considerations of nationality, race, creed, colour, age, sex, politics or social status.

Nurses render health services to the individual, the family and community and coordinate their services with those of related groups.

Nurses and People

The nurse's primary responsibility is to those who require nursing care.

The nurse holds in confidence personal information and uses judgment in sharing this information.

Nurses and Practice

The nurse carries personal responsibility for nursing practice and for maintaining competence by continual learning.

The nurse maintains the highest standards of nursing care possible within the reality of a specific situation.

The nurse uses judgment in relation to individual competence when accepting and delegating responsibilities.

The nurse, when acting in a professional capacity, should at all times maintain standards of personal conduct that would reflect credit upon the profession.

Nurses and Society

The nurse shares with other citizens the responsibility for initiating and supporting action to meet the health and social needs of the public.

Nurses and The Profession

The nurse plays the major role in determining and implementing desirable standards of nursing practice and nursing education.

The nurse is active in developing a core of professional knowledge.

The nurse, acting through the professional organization, participates in establishing and maintaining equitable social and economic working conditions in nursing.

Nurses and Co-Workers

The nurse sustains a cooperative relationship with co-workers in nursing and other fields.

The nurse takes appropriate action to safeguard the individual when his care is endangered by a co-worker or any other person.

AMERICAN MEDICAL ASSOCIATION

PRINCIPLES OF MEDICAL ETHICS

PREAMBLE   These principles are intended to aid physicians individually and collectively in maintaining a
high level of ethical conduct. They are not laws but
standards by which a physician may determine the pro-
priety of his conduct in his relationship with patients,
with colleagues, with members of allied professions,
and with the public.

SECTION 1 The principal objective of the medical profession is to render services to humanity with full respect for the dignity of man. Physicians should merit
the confidence of patients entrusted to their care,
rendering to each a full measure of service and devo-
tion.

SECTION 2 Physicians should strive continually to improve medical knowledge and skill, and should make a-
vailable to their patients and colleagues the benefits
of their professional attainments.

SECTION 3 A physician should practice a method of
healing founded on a scientific basis; and he should
not voluntarily associate professionally with anyone
who violates this principle.

SECTION 4 The medical profession should safeguard the
public and itself against physicians deficient in moral
character or professional competence. Physicians should
observe all laws, uphold the dignity and honor of the
profession and accept its self-imposed disciplines.
They should expose, without hesitation, illegal or unethical conduct of fellow members of the profession.

SECTION 5 A physician may choose whom he will serve.
In an emergency, however, he should render service to
the best of his ability. Having undertaken the care of
a patient, he may not neglect him; and unless he has
been discharged he may discontinue his services only
after giving adequate notice. He should not solicit
patients.

SECTION 6 A physician should not dispose of his services under terms or conditions which tend to interfere
with or impair the free and complete exercise of his
medical judgment and skill or tend to cause a

deterioration of the quality of medical care.

SECTION 7 In the practice of medicine a physician should limit the source of his professional income to medical services actually rendered by him, or under his supervision, to his patients. His fee should be commensurate with the services rendered and the patient's ability to pay. He should never pay nor receive a commission for referral of patients. Drugs, remedies or appliances may be dispensed or supplied by the physician provided it is in the best interests of the patients.

SECTION 8 A physician should seek consultation upon request; in doubtful or difficult cases; or whenever it appears that the quality of medical services may be enhanced thereby.

SECTION 9 A physician may not reveal the confidences entrusted to him in the course of medical attendance, or the deficiencies he may observe in the character of patients, unless he is required to do so by law or unless it becomes necessary in order to protect the welfare of the individual or of the community.

SECTION 10 The honored ideals of the medical profession imply that the responsibilities of the physician extend not only to the individual, but also to society where these responsibilities deserve his interest and participation in activities which have the purpose of improving both the health and the well-being of the individual and the community.

CODE OF ETHICS
THE AMERICAN REGISTRY OF X-RAY TECHNICIANS

In consideration of the granting to me of a Certificate of Registration, or a renewal thereof, by the American Registry of X-Ray Technicians, and my attendant right to use the title "Registered Technician" and its abbreviation, "R.T. (ARXT)" in connection with my name, I do hereby agree to perform the duties of an x-ray technician, whether as a worker, teacher, or supervisor, only under the direction or supervision of a duly qualified Doctor of Medicine. I also agree to conduct myself at all times in a manner appropriate to the dignity of my profession consistent with the Principles of Medical Ethics of the American Medical Association.

I will not act as owner, co-owner, advisor, or employer in connection with any type of enterprise having anything to do with the medical use of x-rays unless it be as an Affiliated Registered Technician and subject to the limitations of such certification. I will not interpret radiographs or fluoroscopic shadows, treat or advise patients as to x-ray diagnosis or treatment; nor will I train students in x-ray technology unless under the direct supervision of a duly qualified Doctor of Medicine who specializes in radiology; and I will abide by this Code of Ethics, and all other present and future Rules and Regulations of the American Registry of X-Ray Technicians, as long as I retain my certificate.

_____

signature

CODE OF ETHICS

IN CONSIDERATION OF THE GRANTING TO ME OF A CERTIFICATE OF REGISTRATION, OR THE RENEWAL THEREOF, AND THE ATTENDANT RIGHT TO USE THE TITLE, "REGISTERED RADIOGRAPHER", AND ITS ABBREVIATION, "R.T. (R) (ARRT)", IN CONNECTION WITH MY NAME, I DO HEREBY AGREE TO PERFORM THE DUTIES OF A RADIOGRAPHER ONLY UNDER THE SUPERVISION OF A PERSON WHOSE QUALIFICATIONS ARE ACCEPTABLE TO THIS REGISTRY; AND TO ABIDE BY ALL THE RULES AND REGULATIONS OF THE AMERICAN REGISTRY OF RADIOLOGIC TECHNOLOGISTS AS THEY APPLY TO MY PROFESSION; AND TO CONDUCT MYSELF IN A MANNER APPROPRIATE TO THE DIGNITY OF MY PROFESSION CONSISTENT WITH THE PRINCIPLES OF MEDICAL ETHICS OF THE AMERICAN MEDICAL ASSOCIATION AND THE CODE OF ETHICS OF THE AMERICAN SOCIETY OF RADIOLOGIC TECHNOLOGISTS.

AMERICAN SOCIETY OF RADIOLOGIC TECHNOLOGISTS

CODE OF ETHICS

Preamble
       This Code of Ethics is to serve as a guide by
which Radiologic Technologists may evaluate their professional conduct as it relates to patients, colleagues,
other members of the allied professions and health care
consumers.

       The Code of Ethics is not law but is intended to
assist Radiologic Technologists in maintaining a high
level of ethical conduct.

       Therefore, in the practice of the profession, we
the members of the American Society of Radiologic Technologists, accept the following principles:

Principle 1
       Radiologic Technologists shall conduct themselves
in a manner compatible with the dignity of their profession.

Principle 2
       Radiologic Technologists shall provide services
with consideration of human dignity and the uniqueness
of the patient, unrestricted by considerations of age,
sex, race, creed, social or economic status, handicap,
personal attributes or the nature of the health problem.

Principle 3
       Radiologic Technologists shall make every effort
to protect all patients from unnecessary radiation.

Principle 4
       Radiologic Technologists should exercise and ac-
cept responsibility for independent discretion and
judgment in the performance of their professional services.

Principle 5
       Radiologic Technologists shall judiciously protect
the patient's right to privacy and shall maintain all
patient information in the strictest confidence.

Principle 6
Radiologic Technologists shall apply only methods of technology founded upon a scientific basis and not accept those methods that violate this principle.

Principle 7
Radiologic Technologists shall not diagnose, but in recognition of their responsibility to the patient, they shall provide the physician with all information they have relative to radiologic diagnosis or patient management.

Principle 8
Radiologic Technologists shall be responsible for reporting unethical conduct and illegal professional activities to the appropriate authorities.

Principle 9
Radiologic Technologists should continually strive to improve their knowledge and skills by participating in educational and professional activities and sharing the benefits of their attainments with their colleagues.

Principle 10
Radiologic Technologists should protect the public from misinformation and misrepresentations.

THE RADIOLOGIC TECHNOLOGIST'S CREED

We believe that every Radiologic Technologist should work under the direct supervision of, and be directly responsible to some member of the Radiological, Medical, Surgical, or Dental profession, such member being generally recognized in his profession as being qualified to do the work attempted.

We are opposed to the so-called schools (whether conducted by professional men or laymen) who urges the attendance of any or all laymen with the promise of speedy preparation and handsome remuneration for their services. In other words, we are opposed to the commercial school.

We believe that the standard for all plate and film work should be established by the professional man doing the work of interpretation, and that it is our duty to qualify ourselves to produce the desired standard.

We believe that no expression of our opinion regarding treatment, diagnosis, or interpretation concerning any patient with whom we work should ever be given to other than the professional man to whom we are responsible.

BIBLIOGRAPHY

Abell, Aaron I., ed. American Catholic Thought on So-
    cial Questions. Indianapolis: Bobbs-Merrill,
    1968.

Ackerknecht, E. W. Short History of Medicine. New
    York: Ronald Press Co., 1955.

Agus, Jacob R. The Vision and the Way: An Interpre-
    tation of Jewish Ethics. New York: Ungar, 1966.

Alford, Robert R. Health Care Politics: Ideological
    and Interest Group Barriers to Reform. Chicago:
    University of Chicago Press, 1975.

Barber, Bernard. "Some Problems of the Sociology of
    Professions" in The Professions in America. ed-
    ited by Kenneth S. Lynn. Boston: Haughton-Mif-
    flin, Deaedalus, 1965, pp. 647-865.

Barnlaund, Dean C. "The Mystification of Meaning:
    Doctor-Patient Encounters". Journal of Medical
    Education 51 (1976): 716-725.

Becker, Howard S. "The Nature of a Profession" in
    Education for the Professions. edited by Nelson
    B. Henry. University of Chicago Press, 1960.

Becker, Howard S., and Geer, Blanche. "Medical Educa-
    tion" in Handbook of Medical Sociology. edited
    by Howard E. Freeman, Sol Levine, and Leo G.
    Reeder. Englewood Cliffs, N.J.: Prentice-Hall,
    1963, pp. 169-86.

Berlant, Jeffery Lionel. Professional Monopoly: A
    study of Medicine in the United States and Great
    Britain. Berkeley: University of California
    Press, 1975.

Catholic Hospital Association. Ethical Issues in
    Nursing: A Proceedings. St. Louis: Catholic
    Hospital Association, 1976.

Chayet, Neil L. "Confidentiality and Privileged Com-
    munication" in New England Journal of Medicine
    275 (1966): 1009-1010.

Christman, Luther P. "Nurse-Physician Communication in the Hospital" in Journal of American Medical Association 194 (1965): 539-44.

Cobb, John B. Theology and Pastoral Care. Philadelphia: Fortress Press, 1977.

Coe, Rodney M. Sociology of Medicine. New York: McGraw-Hill, 1970, p. 91.

Crogg, Sydney H. "Interpersonal Relations in Medical Settings" in Handbook of Medical Sociology, edited by Freeman, Levine, and Reeder. Englewood Cliffs, N.J.: Prentice-Hall, 1963, pp. 241-272.

Curran, Charles. Medicine and Morals. Washington, D.C.: Coprus Books.
_____. Politics, Medicine and Christian Ethics: A Dialogue with Paul Ramsey. Philadelphia: Fortress Press.

_____. Issues in Sexual and Medical Ethics. Notre Dame, Ind.: University of Notre Dame Press.

Dubos, Rene. Mirage of Health: Utopicas, Progress and Biological Change. New York: Harper, 1959.

Ellul, Jacques. The Technological Society. New York: Knopf, 1965.

Englehardt, H. Tristram, Jr. "The Concepts of Health and Disease" in Philosophy and Medicine. 1975.

Evans, Lester, J. The Crisis in Medical Education. Ann Arbor: University of Michigan Press, 1964.

Fagin, Claire, et al. "Can We Bring Order Out of the Chaos of Nursing Education" in American Journal of Nursing 76 (1976): 98-107.

Friedson, Eliot. Professional Dominance: The Social Structure of Medical Care. New York: Atherton Press, 1970.

Freund, Paul A. "The Legal Profession" in The Professions in America, edited by Kenneth S. Lynn. Daedulus, 1965, pp. 35-46.

Fromm, Erich. The Revolution of Hope: Toward a Humanized Technology. New York: Bantam Books, 1968.

Fuchs, Josef. <u>Natural Law: A Theological Investiga-</u><u>tion</u>. New York: Sheed and Ward, 1963.

Goldbrunner, Joseph. <u>Holiness is Wholeness</u>. New York: Pantheon, 1955.

Goldstein, Kurt. "Health as a Value" in <u>New Knowledge</u> <u>in Human Values</u>, edited by Abraham M. Maslow. New York: Harper, 1959.

Haring, Bernard. <u>Medical Ethics</u>. Notre Dame, Ind: Fides Publisher, 1973.

Heydebrand, Wolf V. <u>Hospital Bureaucracy: A Compara-</u><u>tive Study of Organizations</u>. New York: Dunellen, 1973.

Howe, Ruel J. <u>The Miracle of Dialogue</u>. New York: Seabury Press, 1963.

Illich, Ivan D. <u>Medical Nemesis: The Expropriation of</u> <u>Health</u>. New York: Pantheon, 1976.

Kelley, Gerald. <u>Medico-Moral Problems</u>. St. Louis: Catholic Hospital Association, 1958.

Kerner, George C. <u>The Revolution in Ethical Theory</u>. New York: Osford University Press, 1966.

Kneller, George F. <u>The Act and Science of Creativity</u>. New York: Holt, 1965.

Lemerton, Richard. <u>Care of the Dying</u>. London: Pricry Press, 1973.

Lepp, Ignace. <u>Death and Its Mysteries</u>. New York: MacMillian, 1968.

McCabe, Hebert. <u>What is Ethics All About?</u> Washington, D.C.: Corpus Books, 1969.

McHugh, James T. <u>Death, Dying and the Law</u>. Our Sun-day Visitor, 1971.

McMurray, John. <u>Persons in Relation</u>. London: Faber and Faber, 1961.

Milgram, Stanley. <u>Obedience to Authority</u>. New York: Harper and Row, 1974.

Mitford, Jessica. The American Way to Death. New York: Simon and Schuster, 1975.

Niebuhr, H. Richard. The Responsible Self. New York: Harper and Row, 1963.

Nouven, Henri J. Intimacy: Pastoral Psychological Essays. Notre Dame: Ind., Fides Publishing.

Outka, Gene. Agape: An Ethical Analysis. New Haven: Yale University Press, 1972.

Pius, XII. "Prolongation of Life: Allocation to an International Congress of Anesthesiologists" in The Pope Speaks 4:393-398.

Rahner, Karl. On the Theology of Death. New York: Herder and Herder.

Ramsey, Paul. The Patient as Person. New Haven: Yale University Press, 1970.

Simon, Yves. The Tradition of Natural Law. New York: Fordham University Press, 1965.

Smith, Harmon L. Ethics and the New Medicine. Nashville, TN.: Abingdon, 1970.

Spicq, Ceslaus. Agape in the New Testament. 3 vols. St. Louis: B. Herder Book Co., 1963.

Stevens, Rosemary. American Medicine and the Public Interest. New Haven: Yale University Press, 1971.

Teale, A. E. Kantian Ethics. Westport, Conn.: Greenwood Press, 1975.

United States Catholic Conference. Ethical and Religious Directives for Catholic Health Facilities. National Conference of Catholic Bishops, 1971.

Veatch, Robert M., and Branson, Roy. Ethics and Health Policy. Cambridge, Mass.: Ballinger, 1976.

Wise, Carroll A. Pastoral Counseling: Its Theory and Practice. New York: Harper, 1951.

Zumbro Valley Medical Society. Religious Aspects of Medical Care: A Handbook of Religious Practices of all Faiths. Medicine and Religion Committee. St. Louis: Catholic Hospital Association, 1975.